continued . . .

"'Trade craft' refers to a functional yet mythical set of skills every warrior, operator, or operative hopes to develop and master as they execute the duties of their trade; Jason Hanson has forgotten more trade craft than most will ever know. I have read many books and manuals focused on teaching and explaining these skill sets, but few hit the mark as cleanly, as effectively, and as easily digestible as *Spy Secrets That Can Save Your Life*. This book is overflowing with practical knowledge and teaching points that can and will save your life. Navy SEALs study all of the elements from this book, but I was stunned to glean so many secrets of the trade that will now join my bag of tricks on and off the battlefield."

—Rorke Denver, Navy SEAL and *New York Times* bestselling author of *Damn Few*

SPY SECRETS THAT CAN SAVE YOUR LIFE

A Former CIA Officer Reveals Safety and Survival
Techniques to Keep You and Your Family Protected

JASON HANSON

A PERIGEE BOOK

PERIGEE

An imprint of Penguin Random House LLC

375 Hudson Street, New York, New York 10014

SPY SECRETS THAT CAN SAVE YOUR LIFE

ISBN: 978-0-399-17514-5

This book has been registered with the Library of Congress.

First edition: September 2015

PRINTED IN THE UNITED STATES OF AMERICA

10   9   8   7   6   5   4   3   2   1

Text design by Laura K. Corless

Contents

SPY SECRETS
THAT CAN SAVE
YOUR LIFE

Introduction

People often ask me why I joined the CIA. The truth is, when you take a look at my childhood it makes perfect sense. When others were picking up girls, I was running around in the woods with a BB gun (or building a potato launcher out of PVC pipe). I also spent lots of time in the Boy Scouts and eventually became an Eagle Scout. If it had to do with adventure, survival, or being prepared, I was drawn to it. As I grew older, I realized I never wanted a normal desk job, and my first job out of college was as a police officer. Soon after, both the Secret Service and the CIA offered me a job. I figured the CIA would be more exciting so I accepted their offer.

When I joined the CIA in 2003, I never imagined that these same tactics I used as a CIA officer for counterintelligence, surveillance, and protecting agency personnel could be so helpful in everyday civilian life. Because of my top-level training, I am blessed to have many unique skills. I can escape from handcuffs within seconds, pick a lock with ease, hotwire a car, use social engineering to get what I want, and know when someone is telling a lie. I can improvise a weapon, pack a perfect emergency kit, and even disappear off the grid if I need to. I can also determine if I'm being followed, deescalate potentially dangerous encounters with would-be attackers, and keep myself and my family safe, both at home and when traveling. Some of these skills are everyday necessities, while others don't come into play very often and are intended mostly for your "inner spy." But all of them can and do save lives. I'd like to share these skills with you because, even though I pray you will never find yourself in danger, you may be the next person saved by this information.

Since leaving the CIA to become an entrepreneur and raise a family, it has been my mission to share my life-saving tactics with others. My passion for personal safety and security led me to open my training school, Spy Escape and Evasion, in 2010. After several extremely successful years teaching these techniques to thousands of people all around the world, including CEOs, celebrities, security specialists, high-net-worth individuals, stay-at-home moms, and college students, I realized it was time to share this information with as many people as possible who are interested in keeping themselves and their families safe. It is my hope that *Spy Secrets That Can Save Your Life* will show you that you don't have to be an intelligence officer to remain safe in an uncertain world. I have successfully taught my spy escape and evasion techniques to thousands of people through my fun and intensive training courses. My Spy Secrets have helped regular, everyday people thwart kidnappings, stop home invasions, prevent muggings, and avoid carjackings. Here are just a few ways these methods have saved lives:

Amy O. from Virginia knew immediately how to handle herself when she realized she was being followed on a running trail near her home.

Jared L. from Las Vegas knew exactly what to do when he was threatened in an elevator in a parking garage.

Dan P. from Los Angeles shared that after taking my class he was able to avoid harm when an angry and threatening man approached his car near the airport.

Gary S., the vice president of a manufacturing company, who travels eleven months out of the year, avoided two separate mugging attempts in China.

Heather M. from Sarasota, Florida, was able to escape using her tactical pen when two men tried to kidnap her at a gas station.

Dennis R. from Texas was able to survive a violent home invasion by using the tactics taught in my Spy Escape and Evasion course.

These individuals survived potentially dangerous or even life-threatening situations because they knew exactly what to do. They reacted using the various tactics from my courses and avoided becoming victims of violent crimes. It is my goal that after reading this book that you will be empowered and confident, knowing how to respond in any crisis or emergency situation you or your loved ones might face.

SURVIVAL INTELLIGENCE

You're about to acquire some exciting new skills. After reading this book, you'll know how to escape quickly out of duct tape and rope and will know how to tell if someone is lying to you or trying to social engineer you into an unwelcome situation. That being said, the skills you're about to learn need to be accompanied by something equally important—what I call survival intelligence. In short, survival intelligence involves having the confidence to know that you can respond appropriately in any emergency situation. You can react quickly and smartly during a crisis using the tools you have on hand. You're prepared and know you can provide for your family's safety. Because I feel survival intelligence is as important as the skills I'm about to teach you, I've created seven easy-to-follow rules to help you achieve and maintain it. Following these rules will put you in the best position possible to protect yourself and your family.

Throughout the book, you'll be reminded of the importance of these rules, and it's my belief that actively following them can mean the difference between staying safe and facing a tragedy. You'll also note that I've used stories from all over the world to demonstrate how my various tactics can be used. While reading about tragedies or near tragedies that have taken place, you may find yourself wondering, "What were they thinking?" Or "How did they not see that coming?" It's my hope that by following a few critical rules, you and your family will never be in a position where you're asking yourself, "How did we not see that?" but will instead be empowered to act quickly and appropriately in any dangerous situation that comes your way.

Rule 1: Practice Adaptability

Life is rarely completely cut and dry. My intelligence training has taught me that while knowing what to do in emergency situations is important, ultimately it's being adaptable that can save you. As you learn various skills throughout the book, keep in mind that it's *your ability to put them into practice in unexpected situations* that can make the biggest difference. Life doesn't always go as planned, and it's crucial to be ready to tackle what it throws at you with the tools you have on hand. The best part about this rule is that it isn't hard to practice. You'll see that while being a fast, strong, powerful person is great, there's a limit to how helpful this can be if you're unable to adapt to a new and potentially threatening situation. Make a point of cultivating adaptability whenever you can.

Rule 2: Be Self-Reliant

I'm a big believer in self-reliance. I simply don't want to depend on someone else to take care of my family or myself. I think self-reliance and personal responsibility are to be valued. This goes beyond personal philosophy. Throughout the course of this book you're going to be reading about some situations that ended tragically, and unnecessarily so, often due, at least in part, to a lack of self-reliance. It is my hope that everyone who reads this book will see the importance of being able to act for himself or herself in an emergency situation. I believe it is crucial to have both the tools on hand and the ability to act to save yourself if necessary. Our country has faced some challenging times that have tested the self-reliance of many people. For example, terrorist attacks and natural disasters have resulted in many people realizing they must fend for themselves in the aftermath of a crisis. As you'll see in this book, some people were more prepared to do this than others.

Self-Reliance = Helping Others

Make no mistake. While I believe self-reliance is a key trait when it comes to survival, there's another reason it's valuable. When we learn to be self-reliant, we put ourselves in a position to help others. It is my hope that after reading this book, the skills I'm going to teach you combined with a strong sense of self-reliance will put you in a stronger position to be useful to others in an emergency situation.

Rule 3: Don't Be a Hero

Let me be clear. The rule about not being a hero isn't about not taking action and isn't about not being a valued, helpful member of society. This rule is about being a bigger person and having the good sense to walk away from a potential confrontation—even if there is a part of you that doesn't want to. Trust me, I know how hard this can be. I was running early one morning in Baltimore, Maryland, toward the inner harbor. I noticed two guys on the sidewalk ahead of me. I was in my jogging clothes, and they were fully dressed walking around at 6 a.m., which is a bit unusual. As I ran toward them, I saw them look at each other and then spread apart, creating a situation in which I'd have to run between the two of them. Once I was between them, who knows what they were going to do. I decided to play it safe: run across the street, making sure to give them eye contact and let them know I'm paying attention. Maybe it was nothing. Maybe they had six friends around the corner and they were going to rob me. My main point is that I didn't let my ego get in the way; I didn't feel a need to prove myself by running between them (although you'll soon learn why my decision to give them eye contact was important) and risk a potentially dangerous situation.

In another instance, a drunken idiot came out of a gas station and gave me the bird and started telling me off. Turns out, he thought I was someone he knew who had the same car. My response? "No problem. Don't worry about it." I might have wanted to tell this guy off, but I have the sense to know that it's simply not worth it.

I can tell you that the toughest, most highly skilled guys I met while in the CIA were also the quietest. They were confident in their abilities and didn't need to go around boasting about their skills. I'm smart enough to know that it's best to avoid escalation. I don't need to put myself at risk of meeting that one guy who has better skills than I do or someone who happens to get lucky that day. Feel empowered by the skills you have, and the ones I'm going to teach you, but be smart about when you use them.

Rule 4: Movement Saves Lives

This is not the only time you're going to hear me say this: Movement saves lives. As you read about various situations people have been faced with throughout the book, you'll see that it's those who move are the ones who survive. This is also known as getting off of the X. The concept works in a couple of ways, and I'll outline how to handle various scenarios in greater detail in later chapters. To give you the basic idea, think about it this way. If someone comes at you with a knife, you have a couple of immediate choices—you can move out of the way or you can get stabbed. I'm obviously simplifying the situation, but I want you to see that moving when threatened needs to be your first priority. This concept works in other ways too—for example, you may be surprised to learn that many people often survive the impact of a plane crash, but then die from inhaling the toxic smoke. Some people are so shocked by the crash that they can't even manage to unbuckle their seat belts, and they die as a result. The people who aren't killed on impact and make it out alive are the ones who get out of their seats and *move*. They don't freeze. They unbuckle their seat belts and quickly get themselves out of danger. You simply want to remember that in any threatening situation—whether it's a hurricane, a plane crash, or terrorist attack—movement saves lives.

Rule 5: Perception Is Everything

One of the best things about sharing my spy secrets is that some of them are so simple and easy to execute that you can basically put the book down and make a potentially life-saving change in just seconds. This is because perception is important, and I'm going to teach you about the various actions you can take to give off a particular perception—whether it's that you're not a person to be messed with and criminals should stay away or that your house is the one house on the block that a criminal shouldn't dare try to rob. To properly execute the physical and psychological tricks I'm going to show you in this book, you need to start being aware of the perceptions both you and others give off. Ask yourself the following questions: Do I look like a person who would be an easy victim? Does my house appear uninhabited? Am I walking with confidence? What about those around you? Is the person sitting next to you in a restaurant acting suspiciously? Are you being followed by the man who you just passed in the grocery store? Learning to be aware of perceptions can play a key role in remaining safe.

Rule 6: Notice Baselines

Being aware of baselines, or what's normal, is a key concept in most intelligence work. You simply can't know if you're about to walk into an unsafe situation unless you're familiar with what's normal for a particular place. Is this street always so crowded? Is the noise level I'm hearing normal? Or has something happened? If you're not acutely familiar with the baseline of your home, your neighborhood, and your place of employment, you will not be properly equipped to know if you are about to be in harm's way and need to take immediate action. Being able to establish a baseline is a key component for any intelligence work, and I'm going to show how to do this in detail.

Rule 7: Practice Situational Awareness at All Times

This final rule is the cornerstone of my philosophy. No amount of training can keep you safe if you do not practice situational awareness. I feel so strongly about this that I dedicated an entire chapter of this book to practicing situational awareness, and I maintain that my ability to remain situationally aware is the most important thing I learned while in the CIA. The bottom line is that that *nothing I teach you can keep you safe if you're not aware of what's happening around you.* If your nose is buried in your smartphone or you're having a distracting conversation while walking down the street, my tactics for knowing if you're being followed, for example, aren't going to work. Again, you're going to be reading about some senseless tragedies that could have been prevented if situational awareness had been practiced. You'll see that I'm not promoting paranoia—just a healthy sense of what's happening around you. Situational awareness is what enables you to get off the X before you're attacked or to cross the street before you're mugged. It takes practice and some dedication, but it's doable, and it may save your life.

A Safer, Happier Life

My mission in writing *Spy Secrets That Can Save Your Life* and starting the Spy Escape and Evasion training school is to help people live a safer and happier life. These seven rules we've just touched upon, combined with the arsenal of self-defense tactics you're about to learn, will help quell your anxiety. We're living in frightening and unpredictable times, but I believe you should not live in fear. Knowledge, skill, and awareness will give you peace of mind that you can handle any event that might arise.

2

SITUATIONAL AWARENESS

The Single Most Important Thing
I Learned in the CIA

At an upscale Mexican restaurant in Manhattan, workers quickly hid when masked men, one in possession of a machete, robbed the restaurant. One customer at the bar remained completely oblivious to the robbery that was taking place, essentially right in front of him. While the robbers searched behind the bar for cash, this person not only continued to look at his phone, but raised his glass in a manner that indicated he'd like another drink. While he missed the entire robbery, he did actually move over to the next bar stool to make room for one of the robbers to escape. The man later told the detectives that he "did not know what had happened" and had been "staring at his phone the entire time." Managing to miss a robbery that's happening right around you shows an amazing lack of what's known as *situational awareness*.

People are often surprised when I tell them the most important thing I learned in the CIA is situational awareness. CIA officers receive the best possible self-defense training in how to ward off any kind of attack, how to escape restraints in seconds, and what to do in a car chase—but ultimately it's situational awareness that's going to keep an officer alive. We also know that it's best to completely avoid any kind of violent confrontation. It's our knowledge of situational awareness that allows us to act *before* a crisis occurs. If guns are drawn, it's because we missed something, and our situational awareness was lacking.

I've also experienced firsthand how important this skill is as a civilian. I met my wife while she was in law school in Baltimore. Her school was in a transitional area. While it wasn't extremely dangerous, it was on the sketchy side, and someone had recently been stabbed on a bridge near the school. I didn't want her walking around alone after night classes, and I always made a point of picking her up. But it turns out that we encountered trouble in broad daylight. It was a gorgeous fall day, so I decided to meet my wife and take her to lunch in Baltimore's inner harbor. Right on the water, the inner harbor is full of shops and restaurants, and it's one of the nicer spots the city has to offer. As we were walking to the inner harbor, I noticed a man behaving very suspiciously. He had crossed the street in front of us several times, and he was giving me a ton of eye contact, really staring me down. The man settled about two feet away from where I was standing. While my wife and I were waiting for the walk signal so that we could cross the street, he stood directly to my left. Because he was giving me so much eye contact, I was watching him in my peripheral vision, and paying a lot of attention to what he was doing. I made a point of watching his hands. It's hands that kill—hands reach for knives or guns and throw punches. When the light turned, I purposely started taking small steps. I noticed that the guy was pacing me, walking step for step with me. At this point I had my tactical pen out. After about three steps, I turned to him and I said, "Excuse me, do you know what time it is?" He looked at me funny, and I said again, "Excuse me, do you know what time it is?" He responded, "Four-thirty." We stared at each other for about a second, but it felt like an eternity. Suddenly he turned around and quickly walked away. He crossed the street and I never saw him again.

By asking him what time it was, I accomplished two things. First, I had completely removed the element of surprise. My hands were up, so if necessary I could strike or disarm him. Secondly, I know that a normal reaction time is approximately one and a half seconds. That's how long, at minimum, it takes a person to react to a situation. I knew that if he attacked, I'd need one and half seconds to do what was necessary to protect myself and my wife. The guy proceeded to tell me the time and immediately turned around and walked the other way (the fact that he then changed direction is a sure sign he was planning to do something). If this guy were innocent, he would have kept walking to the inner harbor like he was originally.

Criminals don't want their targets to know they're onto them, but I knew. And by indicating to him that I knew what was going on, he made a choice to move on. Practicing situational awareness put me in a position to know that something was off. By being alert to my surroundings, I was able to identify that my wife and I were in harm's way, and I was able to take action. While there are many ways this situation could have been defused, the important thing was that I did *something*. I trusted my gut and reacted. Had I been paying attention to my cell phone instead of what was happening around me, I would have ended up in an altercation with a mugger.

What Is Situational Awareness?

If you take a look at what most people are doing on the street, at a playground, or a shopping mall, you're going to see one common factor. The majority of people are either talking on their phones, or sending and reading text messages. If you are looking at your phone, you have your head down, you're disengaged, and you likely have no idea what's actually going on around you. Or maybe you're not talking on your cell phone, but you're preoccupied by work, stress, or just daydreaming about an upcoming vacation. The bottom line is that if you're not alert and aware, you are vulnerable. There are many situations in which injury (or worse) could have been avoided if people

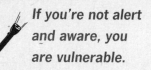 *If you're not alert and aware, you are vulnerable.*

were practicing situational awareness. In San Francisco, there was a rash of cell phone users being assaulted and robbed in public. A forty-three-year-old man was punched and robbed while texting in broad daylight on a crowded street corner. An up-and-coming comedian in New York fell onto the subway tracks while texting and was struck by a train. Miraculously she survived. A fifteen-year-old girl in the San Diego area was less fortunate. She was standing on a street corner texting when she attempted to cross against the light. Her brother tried to stop her, but he was too late. She stepped into the path of an oncoming truck and was killed. Had any of these individuals been paying attention to their immediate surroundings, these tragic situations would have been avoided.

Smartphones and Situational Awareness

I realize this might sound weird, but I've never sent a text message in my entire life, and I have no plans to. While smartphones may have some great features, I think they are terrible for situational awareness. How many times have you been stopped at a green light and the guy in front of you was too busy texting to notice the light was now green? The bottom line is that none of my training as a CIA officer is going to help me if I'm too busy texting to notice I'm in danger. There are other reasons I stick to a flip phone—smartphones store too much personal information, and they can suck up too much time—but the main reason is that smartphones are simply a threat to my situational awareness.

The Most Important Colors: White, Yellow, Orange, and Red

At its most basic, situational awareness is about remaining alert and knowing what's going on around you. It's really about being able to assess your environment, anticipating danger, and being ready to take any further action if necessary. What I recommend following, and what I teach in my Spy Escape and Evasion courses, are the Cooper Color Codes. These are four stages of readiness that enable a person to be in a mind-set to react appropriately and quickly to a threat.

Jeff Cooper was a Marine who served in the Pacific on the USS *Pennsylvania* during World War II. Cooper returned to active duty during the Korean War, where he was promoted to lieutenant colonel. In the 1970s, Cooper founded the American Pistol Institute in Arizona, where he taught handgun and rifle classes to civilians as well as law enforcement and military personnel. While Cooper was known for his handgun and firearm expertise, he also believed that actual weapons or self-defense skills did not provide the best way to survive a potentially fatal attack. Cooper believed that the most effective tool was a person's mind-set. Cooper's Color Codes are used to describe different degrees of situational awareness, as follows:

Condition White: Unprepared and totally unaware. The individuals I described earlier in this chapter would have been operating under Condition White. It is crucial that you learn to avoid this condition at all times.

What it looks like: Head down, eyes averted, oblivious to what's going on around you. A person in Condition White may be daydreaming, talking on a cell phone, texting, or engaged in a conversation. If you're in Condition White you may be sitting on a bench reading or you might walk into a dark alleyway at night without thinking twice about it, putting yourself in a position where you could easily be attacked. If you aren't alert to what's happening in your immediate environment, you are vulnerable and unprepared for whatever might happen next.

Condition Yellow: Relaxed alert. When you are in Condition Yellow, there's no specific threat, but you remain alert and aware. Condition Yellow isn't about expecting an attack but about allowing yourself to be constantly taking in information about what's going on around you. People functioning in Condition Yellow are difficult to surprise. This is how most people operated before cell phones.

What it looks like: Your head is up, you're aware of your surroundings. You may be having a conversation, but aren't so distracted that you wouldn't notice a car coming your way, or a person heading toward you with intent to attack. A person in Condition Yellow would definitely notice a strange person approaching him on the street, and would have ample time to decide how to respond—by crossing the street, changing direction, calling for help, and so on. Condition Yellow allows you to notice if trouble is coming your way. It's important to remember that staying in condition yellow keeps you out of Condition Red, which I'll get to in a minute. Being in Condition Yellow while walking with my wife in Baltimore City is what kept us from getting mugged, and it can help you stay safe too.

Condition Orange: A state in which there is a specific alert. You may notice a man in a thick winter coat walking around a crowded building in the middle of August. You may be walking to the parking lot when you notice someone paying too much attention to you. Something about a situation or an individual feels potentially threatening. You prepare yourself by putting your hand on your tactical pen or you get out your cell phone to call for help.

What it looks like: I immediately went into Condition Orange when my wife and I were standing on the street next to the person I believed was going to harm us. I was in Condition Yellow (aware) when I noticed something off about this particular person. Once in Condition Orange, I got out my tactical pen. (I always carry a gun where I legally can, but I don't have a concealed carry permit for the state of Maryland. I'll get to the benefits of carrying a tactical pen shortly.) I remained alert and was ready to deflect an attack. If you feel a person is following you, turning around and walking into a crowded store is another example of a Condition Orange response.

Condition Red: Condition Red is the crisis condition, but you are mentally prepared to fight or escape. You've predetermined what exactly was going to cause you to react, and you've now received that specific trigger from the criminal. You got out your tactical pen while you were still in Condition Orange, but now you're striking your attacker with it, fighting for your life. While it's entirely possible the situation may involve fighting or using a weapon or any self-defense tactics you have, it's also possible the situation will be resolved by other means such as calling 911 or running into a well-populated area.

What it looks like: A person is responding to a real threat. She has predetermined that this threat is likely to occur, and has not been taken by complete surprise. This individual in Condition Red may have already noted an escape and is running to it, has decided to thwart off the attacker, may have drawn a knife or other weapon, or may be calling for help.

Stay in Yellow to Avoid Red

Heather, who is a graduate of my Spy Escape and Evasion course, avoided a carjacking because she was practicing good situational awareness. "When I'm at the gas station, I always remember what I learned in Jason's class," she reports. "Keep your keys in your hand, *not* your phone, and be aware of what's going on around you. I was nearly finished pumping gas when I saw a man running up to me on my right side. He seemed to be coming out of the woods behind the gas station. He was shouting, 'Excuse me!' very loudly, trying to get my attention. I also noticed there was a second man approaching. My gut told me something was very wrong, and I was glad I had my tactical pen on me. I screamed at him and told him to back off. I put the pump down, and drove off. They both lunged toward my car. I was convinced they wanted the car—and if they had the car, they had me too."

Because Heather was operating in Condition Yellow, she was able to immediately determine that this person wanted to do her harm. She was able to see right away that the potential carjacker was working with someone else. She was aware, and therefore did not fall for the criminals' plan to distract her while the other person came up to her from behind. Had Heather allowed herself to be distracted by the first man, she could have lost her car, or worse, her life.

While making an effort to operate on Condition Yellow takes some getting used to, it's a simple change that could ultimately save your life. Choosing to put away the cell phone and walk down the street with your head up is a big start, but you'll also want to sharpen your senses. Your gut will often tell you when something is wrong, and it's important to listen, but there are some additional strategies that can help you be more aware if danger is looming.

Get Off the *X*: The Most Important Thing to Remember in Any Emergency

In addition to practicing good situational awareness, it is critical you remember the one simple concept that can keep you from being injured or worse. In the event you are faced with a life-and-death situation of any kind, you need *to move*. I'll be referring to this frequently throughout the book, when I say, "Get off the *X*." You'll see in the stories I tell that *people who move live*. It's freezing and staying put that will get you injured or even killed. If someone is headed directly at you with a knife, getting off the *X* and moving will prevent you from being stabbed. Similarly, leaving town in time to avoid a major storm is getting 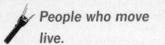 **People who move live.** off the *X*. It's essential that you remember that movement saves lives.

It Did *Not* Come Out of Nowhere: Recognizing Pre-Incident Indicators

Many victims will tell you they had no idea they were about to be attacked. The truth is, there are clear-cut signs most criminals exhibit before attacking someone. When my wife and I were headed to our lunch in Baltimore, you'll remember I noticed the man was giving me intense eye contact and matched our pacing. These are known as *pre-incident indicators*. Pre-incident indicators can be described as predictable patterns of behavior that a person will exhibit in a particular situation. There are several recognizable pre-incident indicators that can alert you to potential criminal be-havior.

Pre-Incident Indicator 1: Staring

Criminals will stare at you for an uncomfortable period of time if they've targeted you for an attack. If you notice a person staring at you for an unnaturally long period of time, cross the street, ask for help, or do whatever it takes to get out of their way. The reason they stare at you is because they've locked eyes on their target, and that target is you. The criminal has made the decision to go after you, and when a predator finds his prey he keeps his eyes on it.

Pre-Incident Indicator 2: Pacing

Only people with ill intent will match your pacing. It is not natural for humans to want to walk in step with strangers, so be aware when someone is matching your pace. This is also true in vehicles. If you and another vehicle are driving side by side on the highway, one car will speed up or slow down. You will notice that if you vary your speed, the criminal will walk slower or faster to match your stride. This indicates that you need to get away from this person and to safety as quickly as possible.

Pre-Incident Indicator 3: Distraction

Heather from my Spy Escape and Evasion class did not allow her-self to be distracted by a man coming at her shouting, "Excuse me!" She saw his ploy for what it was—a distraction. Criminals will often work in pairs or groups, with one person distracting the victim with a question, plea for help, or even an offer of help if you appear lost or are obviously a stranger to an area. Once you are distracted, the other criminal will have a perfect opening to steal your purse, wallet, or phone, or worse.

Beating Normalcy Bias: Knowing That It *Can* Happen to You

To this day, Penelope regrets getting on the subway during the September 11 attacks. "I lived right on the water, and had a perfect view of the twin towers. I walked out of my apartment building in Brooklyn and saw flames and smoke pouring out of a hole in one of the towers. Obviously something horrible had happened. Lots of people were gathering around and watching. Someone said a small plane had crashed into the towers. I was immediately comforted by this. It made *sense*." Even though she was shaken by what she saw, Penelope decided it was probably an accident, so she got on the subway and continued to work as normal. It was when she was on the subway that it became clear that something terrible was going on, and that she had put herself in a very unsafe position. "There was an announcement that a second plane had hit the World Trade Center. I immediately knew something big was happening and I was very scared. I didn't know what was going on, but it seemed like a good idea to get off the subway and walk away from the towers immediately." Penelope was fortunate that she was not directly in harm's way as so many other people were that day, but she likely would have made different choices had she not be impacted by what's known as *normalcy bias*.

Normalcy bias is how humans cope with unwanted change. It's a way of processing traumatic events or disasters. Humans are wired to fear change. When a big event is about to take place or is taking place, such as a hurricane, terrorist attack, or an outbreak of an illness, it's natural for us to try to normalize the situation to the best of our ability. As Penelope puts it, "In a million years I never would have assumed we were being attacked by terrorists. A terrorist attack just wasn't in my realm of possibility. My brain simply did not process this."

While normalcy bias is a protective mechanism, it's something we must learn to combat and be aware of to stay safe. It's normalcy bias that allows us to think that we're going to be OK, or an approaching storm isn't going to be that bad. This is how normalcy bias puts us in danger. If we aren't aware of the impact a particular event may have, we're not able to adequately prepare for it. Left unchecked, normalcy bias can lead us into dangerous behaviors, such as these:

1. **Not taking a disaster seriously:** If you don't recognize how deadly a storm or potential terrorist attack can be, you will not be prepared when such an event occurs. You may do something that puts you at further risk. For instance, Penelope would have been safer staying home than riding the subway into lower Manhattan. Had she taken the situation more seriously, she would have been aware that going into Manhattan was risky.

2. **Not preparing for a disaster:** We've all seen how crowded Home Depot gets the night before a big snow-storm. People are out buying shovels, salt, or whatever is needed. The same could be said for other disasters. In certain parts of the country, people routinely experience hurricanes or wildfires. Yet, not all of these people will prepare properly by planning escape routes and having supplies and food on hand. Normalcy bias keeps people from planning appropriately. They may think, "The fire will never reach this far, so I don't need to prepare." Or "I'll be rescued if there's ever a real problem."

3. **Believing that because something hasn't happened before, it never will:** It's hard to know how to react when dealing with a new experience. People who are hindered by normalcy bias tend to stay positive and not acknowledge that just because something hasn't hap-pened before, doesn't mean it can't. As we've seen in just the past few years, terrorist attacks, hurricanes, torna-dos, and blizzards do happen—and not always when and where you'd expect. While I'm not suggesting you spend all of your time worrying about every situation that could possibly happen, it is important to not let normalcy bias get in the way of your being a prepared individual. Nor-malcy bias isn't just about being prepared for a storm or other disaster. It's really a state of mind that you have to learn to manage in order to practice good situational awareness.

I Didn't Know, I Saw: Secrets to Establishing a Baseline

How do you determine whether a seemingly normal situation is starting to turn dangerous? How can you pick up subtle cues that something is off—that a situation isn't quite what it seems? Establishing a baseline is key to knowing whether a situation is potentially dangerous. Establishing a baseline requires that you note significant or subtle changes occurring in a particular place or in a person's behavior. The BBC's modern take on the character Sherlock Holmes presents one of the best (but extreme) examples of a person who can quickly and accurately gather information about a person. When Sherlock meets Watson for the first time, he casually asks him "Iraq or Afghanistan?" Based on Watson's answer (Afghanistan) and spending literally only a few seconds with him, Sherlock is able to determine that Watson is an injured war doctor, that Watson sees a therapist, and that his therapist believes his limp is psychosomatic. Watson quite naturally is stunned by Sherlock's accuracy. When Watson asks Sherlock how he knew, Sherlock replies, "I didn't know, I saw."

He goes on to explain, "Your haircut, the way you hold yourself, says military. The conversation as you entered the room said trained at Bart's, so army doctor. Obvious. Your face is tanned, but no tan above the wrists—you've been abroad but not sunbathing. The limp's really bad when you walk, but you don't ask for a chair when you stand, like you've forgotten about it, so it's at least partly psychosomatic. That suggests the original circumstances of the injury were probably traumatic—wounded in action, then. Wounded in action, suntan—Afghanistan or Iraq."

What Exactly Is a Baseline?

You can be operating on Condition Yellow, aware of what's happening around you, but if your brain isn't allowing you to see, or register and react to, what's normal or not normal, you won't be able to take appropriate measures to stay safe. To determine what is normal—whether it be for a particular person or a place, you need to take a baseline. A baseline is an informal measure that determines what is normal and what is not. A close friend who tells you, "Hey, you're looking really good these days" is able to make that comparison because he knows what you look like on a day-to-day basis—he knows your baseline. He'll be able to notice if you've gotten some sun or are looking especially well rested. If a child who usually has a robust appetite suddenly isn't hungry at dinner, you may think something is off. She may be getting sick, or maybe she just had too many after-school snacks. Of course, for another child this might be normal—and if he started eating much more than he usually does, you would think something was amiss. These are very basic examples of everyday baselines, circumstances in which someone is aware of what is typical and what isn't in a given situation. It's important to note that these are not universal norms; rather they are specific to our situation and surroundings.

Places Have Baselines Too

As you may expect, almost all major government buildings have fence lines with cameras and alarms that go off in some type of operations center. Cameras now play a critical role in maintaining a facility's security by establishing the baseline for the actual building. The camera's sensors pick up bits of information and are able to determine what is normal on the fence line on an average day. If something out of the ordinary occurs, like a deer or a person approaches the fence line, the operations center would immediately be notified. The cameras know the baseline; the cameras know when something different happens. In a similar way, you can make a point of knowing when something is off of your baseline. Would you know immediately upon arriving home if something was different? Would you be able to tell if a potentially dangerous event was occurring near your office? Establishing a baseline of your home, your immediate surroundings, and places you frequent can save your life.

Marie knew immediately that something was wrong when she opened the door to her apartment. "A plant on the desk had been knocked over. I knew I hadn't knocked over that plant." Marie immediately noticed a few other things that were off. "We had a container in the living room that held our change. It was tipped on its side. I also saw that the window was open. I was positive the window was closed when I left in the morning." Marie knew the baseline of her apartment. She made a point of closing the windows every time she left the building, and was positive the plant and change were out of place. Her awareness of what was normal for her apartment was off. She knew someone had been in the apartment and she immediately called the police. Unfortunately, not everyone is in tune with his or her baseline as Marie. An Orlando, Florida, woman was lucky to remain physically unharmed after two separate robberies. Lisa Bailey and her son Ryan returned home to find their garage door open. Ryan believed he had left the garage door open before leaving for school that day. The family walked into the house to discover their computer and television were missing, the cabinets and drawers were all open, and food was even removed from the refrigerator. In a later incident, the family came home to find a black Jeep with a crying toddler in the backseat parked in their driveway. Rather than call the police, Ms. Bailey walked in on burglars. The criminals were climbing out the back window as she was entering her home. This family is incredibly fortunate that despite their failure to notice that their baseline was off, they were not hurt or even killed by the burglars.

Know Your Norm—And Keep It Consistent

To stay safe, it's important to familiarize yourself with baselines. By establishing a baseline for your home and other places you frequent, you will be able to sense immediately when something isn't right. Marie knew right away that someone had been in her home, because she knew and maintained a baseline. It's crucial to have a solid, preplanned security routine in place. Make sure this is followed every time you leave the house. While the specifics of your security routine must reflect the needs of your family and home, be sure to include the following in your routine:

- Lock all doors.
- Close and lock all windows.
- Shut and lock the garage.
- Turn on/off exterior lighting.

You should also be sure you and your family members are aware of other procedures. Do you shut all blinds or curtains before going out? Were lights left on? If your family discusses normal procedures before leaving the house, each member of your family will immediately be able to determine if the baseline is off. Remember, if you ever think someone is in your home, do not attempt to enter. The risk to your own safety is not worth it. Call the police.

What Does Experience Tell You?

Just like you should know if something is wrong with the baseline of your home, you should also be able to tell if something is off when shopping, going to work, or you're at your child's school. It's not unusual to be watching the news or reading an article where someone says, "I knew something was wrong." People who are in tune with the baseline of their surroundings are able to pick up on the sometimes subtle (but not always) clues that something is wrong. These people not only understand what a baseline should look like but they're also not letting normalcy bias get in the way. Erin Sarris, a runner who survived the Boston Marathon bombing knew something was wrong. "I didn't know what it was, but I knew it wasn't thunder, because it was a beautiful day with just some high, puffy clouds." Sarris got out her cell phone immediately, connected with her husband and got out of the area. She soon saw lots of ambulances approaching and her suspicions were confirmed. Sarris knew that a loud noise that was not related to the weather signaled a potentially dangerous situation. Katherine Walton, a thirty-nine-year-old American, was shopping at a mall in Nairobi with her five children when a brutal terrorist attack occurred. She recalled hearing "very loud explosions" and immediately knew something was wrong. She was able to hide with three of her children, and texted the other two to stay hidden until the danger had passed. In both of these cases, the women reacted. They did not wait to see what was going on, or make the assumption that even though they had heard something highly unusual, that things must be OK. They did not let normalcy bias get in the way. To determine whether a situation may potentially be dangerous, ask yourself the following key question:

Based on what I know from past experience, does everything appear as it should?

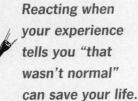

Reacting when your experience tells you "that wasn't normal" can save your life.

If a situation appears different from what you know to be normal, you need to consider the possibility that something might be wrong. Reacting when your experience tells you "that wasn't normal" can save your life.

It Starts with Standard Human Behavior

While we can't all have Sherlock Holmes's powers of deduction, we can learn something from his unusual abilities to make determinations about a person. I'm not suggesting you should be able to figure out where a person lives and works just by looking at him, but knowing how to use small details to learn about a person or situation is important. While we're taught to appreciate each other's differences, we all know that there is a range of behavior that is believed to be acceptable. Behavior can fall anywhere on the spectrum from common to unusual to unacceptable. Human behavior is also influenced by a variety of other factors such as culture, values, and attitudes. What may be viewed as acceptable in one place may be unacceptable in another. It may be perfectly appropriate to wear a suit and tie to work at a law firm, but it would seem extremely strange to show up in a suit if you were a construction worker. It's appropriate to shout and yell at a sporting event, but inappropriate at a play. While standard human behavior may change depending on where the behavior takes place, we all know in our gut if someone's behavior is out of the ordinary and we need to proceed with caution.

Roxanna Ramirez, a twenty-two-year-old Target employee, is credited with saving a seven-year-old child who had been abducted in Pittsburg, California. Ramirez noticed a shopper behaving strangely. "He was fidgeting around, acting really weird, like abnormal. It just didn't make me feel comfortable," she recalled. Ramirez watched the man, and even approached him to ask if he needed any help. She continued to watch him after he left the store, and saw that he continued to behave strangely in his car. Ramirez decided to call the police. Forty-five minutes later the police had a forty-three-year-old man in custody, and Natalie Calvo of Antioch, California, was safe. Clearly Ramirez had observed the man exhibiting something other than standard human behavior. She described him as fidgety and called his behavior weird. In her gut, she knew something was wrong. Because Ramirez was observant and took action, a little girl was saved from a kidnapper. I'm not suggesting you call the police every time you encounter a person who is a bit out of the ordinary, but it's crucial to be aware of what is and is not considered standard human behavior. A few things to consider are the following:

- Is a person dressed inappropriately for the weather? Wearing a winter coat even though it's warm?
- Is the person displaying odd gestures or mannerisms?
- Is the person somewhere he or she isn't supposed to be?
- Is the individual paying too close attention to you or someone else?
- Does the person appear to be following someone?
- Is the person looking around nervously? In other words, is his or her head on a swivel?

Don't Give Criminals the Opportunity

Criminals are often interviewed in prison, shown pictures of people on the street, and asked which ones they'd target. After reading this chapter, it should be no surprise that the victims the criminals chose were the ones operating in Condition White—heads down, talking on the phone, not aware of their surroundings. We only have to look out on the street to know that 99 percent of people have their heads buried in their smartphones. Rarely do we see a person actively paying attention to his surroundings. The good news is that if you practice the tactics we just discussed, and you walk confidently in Condition Yellow with your head up and hands empty, there's little chance that you will become a criminal's next victim, because the criminal will choose an easier target—someone who's not paying attention.

3

YOUR SPY ESCAPE AND EVASION KIT

Crucial Items and Information for Surviving Disasters Both Major and Minor

I believe knowledge is the most important tool of all. That being said, there are situations where some supplies and a few tools can save your life. The world is unpredictable, and I like to approach it prepared for anything. You don't have to comb through history very far to see that being armed with some simple tools can make the difference between life and death. Crime, accidents, and natural disasters can instantly plunge us into danger.

David and Yvonne Higgins were not planning to spend two days trapped in their SUV with their five-year-old daughter. The family was traveling from Texas to a ski resort in New Mexico when they were caught in the middle of a severe snowstorm. The family tried to follow in the tracks of a snowplow, but they soon lost visibility completely. The SUV fell down an embankment and was quickly buried completely by snow. Ms. Higgins described their situation as being "encased in a vehicle igloo." All they could see or feel around them was snow. They huddled together in their ski gear and survived on water and snacks they had packed for the trip. Eventually the trio began to struggle for air. The Higgins family was lucky: They survived and were found in a dramatic search-and-rescue operation that began after Mr. Higgins was able to use his cell phone to contact his brother.

In Atlanta, no one could have imagined that just a couple of inches of snow would render the city helpless. Commuters found themselves trapped in cars for three hours or more, and many ended up abandoning them on the side of the road. Children were trapped at schools when their parents were unable to navigate the massive traffic jams that were happening throughout the city. While in general, the situations I just described ended pretty well, there are times where being caught unprepared has tragic results.

Debbie Este and her teenage daughters in Baton Rouge weren't especially concerned about the coming hurricane. Ms. Este, who recounted her ordeal to CNN, basically expected wind and rain, and then the storm would blow over. They survived the storm unscathed, but after the levees broke, it quickly became clear that the family was in trouble. Within just a few minutes, the water was waist deep. Tiffany, sixteen, lost her cell phone while trying to save a hamster. Her mother rushed into her room to get her credit cards. They found one gallon of drinking water for four people (Ms. Este's sixty-eight-year-old mother was also there). They managed to escape into the attic, which was miraculous, considering Ms. Este had been in a wheelchair for three years. The water made it all the way up to the fifth rung of the ladder that led to the attic. The next day, the water began to seep onto the attic floor, sending the family back into the corner of the dark, windowless space (it had one small air vent). The family had no food, no way to contact anyone, and a very limited water supply. Tragically, Ms. Este's mother, who had suffered congestive heart failure, did not survive. The others were saved when Ms. Este's brother arrived by boat. They were incredibly lucky. Many others lost their lives due to lack of preparedness during Hurricane Katrina, while others survived the storm but did not survive the aftermath.

These stories illustrate an important point—you never know where or when you're going to be faced with a life-or-death situation. Could you and your family survive in your house should you be trapped and unable to get food or water from outside sources? How long could you survive if something goes horribly wrong

You never know where or when you're going to be faced with a life-or-death situation.

while you're out for a drive? And while it's easy to come up with countless examples of weather putting people in peril, there are many other dangerous situations that can occur at a moment's notice.

The Three Tiers of Survival Gear: What an Ex-CIA Officer Really Carries Around

People tend to have some unusual ideas about what intelligence officers carry around, and I wish the truth were half as interesting. People usually expect crazy gadgets—James Bond style, like watches with rotating saws, listening devices hidden in pens, or better yet, a rocket launcher that's concealed inside of a cigarette. While I think my laptop bag has a few things the average person doesn't carry around, it isn't full of gold sovereigns and doesn't launch a throwing knife if you hit the latch a certain way. I've never carried around a bottle of talcum powder that's actually full of tear gas, either. The good news is that many of the items I personally carry are inexpensive, easy to transport, and may save your life. I've divided the gear I carry into three tiers so that you can easily decide what items would work best for you.

Tier One: Everyday Gear

Everyday gear is what I carry on my body, typically in my pockets.

Pocketknife: I like to carry my pocketknife clipped onto the front of my pants pocket where I can access it easily. I usually carry a Benchmade knife, but there are a lot of solid knife makers these days. While a folding knife in your pocket or purse is a must-have item for self-defense and survival, hopefully you'll end up using it only to cut open boxes and packages of hot dogs.

Gun: I carry concealed every day wherever I legally can. Because I love guns you might find me carrying all types such as a Glock 19, Springfield 1911, or Sig Sauer P226 on my hip. I also often carry a Ruger LCP in my right front pocket. It's obviously essential to have proper licensing and training, including training on safe operation and storage, before carrying a firearm. Gun ownership is a serious responsibility that should not be taken lightly.

A cell phone: This is just common sense, as you need to be able to keep in touch. Again, I'm not a fan of smartphones or text messages. I think they interfere with situational awareness, plus it's so easy to get your identity stolen from your smartphone. I believe cell phones are for phone calls. I don't want to be caught off guard when reading a message on the street or while in my car—but I do want to be able to call 911 if needed, and you should too.

Bobby pins: This may sound strange, but I'm going to show you how a simple, inexpensive bobby pin can get you out of some serious situations. I always make sure I have a bobby pin in my Escape & Evasion Gun Belt (CovertBelt.com). It's light as a feather, and you'll never notice it's there.

Monkey's fist paracord keychain: Paracord (sometimes called 550 cord or parachute cord) has many amazing uses. It's incredibly strong and can get you out of some serious jams, which we'll talk about soon. The monkey fist is also a good self-defense tool because it's paracord surrounding a ball bearing that can do some serious damage if you strike someone with it. You can get a free monkey's fist keychain by visiting my website (SpyEscape.com).

Handcuff key: I always keep a handcuff key on my keychain and in my Escape & Evasion Gun Belt. You never know when this might be useful, and it's an item that's allowed on flights, so you don't have to worry about TSA trying to take it away.

American dollars: Cash is king. While the American dollar isn't worth as much as it used to be, I know some guys who have gotten out of some dicey situations thanks to a few twenties or a hundred dollar bill. If you're traveling abroad, and you need to escape out of the back entrance of someone's business—slipping him some cash is going to get you out.

You never know when you're going to need to grease someone's palm, or desperately need a ride to some other location
(normally I wouldn't recommend getting in a car with a
stranger—I'm talking about extreme circumstances), so just
make a point of always carrying some cash with you.

Tactical pen: The tactical pen is one of my all-time favorite
self-defense tools and I'm never without one. The tactical
pen is an appropriate tool for everyone and anyone. At first
glance, it's an actual pen. You can write with it, and it takes
refillable ink from your local office supply store. When you're
not using it to make a list or to write a note, you can use it
to stop an attacker. Thousands of people I've trained carry
tactical pens, ranging from college students to government
workers to overseas travelers. Tactical pens are made out of
aircraft grade aluminum and have a strong pointed end. The
pointed end could be used to stop an attacker and to break
a car window if you've had an accident and need to get out
before your car goes underwater. I also know from my training how much it hurts to get hit with a tactical pen. If you're
being attacked, a sharp jab with this pen in the eyes, kidney
or groin is going to give you an opportunity to escape. I'll
go into more detail about how to use a tactical pen when we
talk about self-defense, but if you want to see the one I use,
visit TacticalSpyPen.com.

Another reason I'm a big fan of the tactical pen is that
you can take them anywhere. You'll have no problem getting
on a plane or into a courthouse with one (I took mine into
the courthouse when going to pay a ticket). Recently, someone who took my course got in touch to let me know that he

got his tactical pen through Ben Gurion Airport in Israel, which is considered the safest airport in the world. It's also a great tool for runners. I like to run myself, and I know many people who feel very comfortable running with a tactical pen. You'd look scary running down the street with a knife in your hand—or a gun (which would be illegal)—but with a tactical pen, no one is going to think twice about it.

Lock pick set: I always carry a lock pick set. I want to be prepared should I end up in a situation where I need to escape a locked room. Plus, it comes in handy for needing access to filing cabinets, locked drawers, or when your neighbors lock themselves out of the house and need your help. They're also easy to get through TSA. In fact, 90 percent of the time I get my set through no problem; about 5 percent of the time a TSA employee will comment on my set, and tell me "it's cool." The other 5 percent of the time they inspect it and give it right back to me. To see the credit card lock pick set I use, visit SafeHomeGear.com. Also, while lock pick sets are legal in most states, be sure to check your state laws before you start carrying one.

Credit card knife: The credit card knife is a great option for people who don't feel comfortable clipping a knife to their clothing. I know many women who prefer a credit card knife to a regular knife. Just like it sounds, the credit card knife is an ingenious knife designed to fold up into the shape of a credit card for safe and easy transportation. The blade pops out of the center of the card, and each side folds back and clips into place. What starts out as a simple "credit card" in your wallet is suddenly a sharp knife that can defend your life or help out in a survival situation. To get a free credit card knife and to watch a video of how the knife works, visit SpyEscape.com.

Tier Two: Laptop Bag Gear or Purse Gear

I'm a busy person. I write articles for various magazines, meet with clients, and teach a lot of classes. When I'm out and about, I have my laptop with me so that I can always get some work done. There are a few essential things I like to keep in my laptop bag along with my materials for work.

Bulletproof panel: Bulletproof panels can come in really handy and actually have a few uses. My bulletproof panel is level 3A, the same material that's used for the bulletproof vests worn by police officers. Level 3A is the highest protection you can get to protect yourself from blunt trauma, and this is what you want in a high-risk situation. In the event there's an active shooter, I'm going to be able to use the panel to protect my vital areas—and my life could be saved. I also use the panel when loading and unloading my gun. I'll just put the muzzle of the gun against the panel, and then I know I have a safe backstop. It works great for dry fire practice as well, as an extra precaution. (You can see a video of my testing the bulletproof panel at Bulletproof Panel.com.)

Spare ammunition: Obviously you need to know what's legal to carry. Where it's legal, I like to carry fifty rounds of ammunition in my laptop bag. The ammo I use is jacketed hollow point rounds, more specifically, Speer Gold Dot.

Lock pick kit: As you know, I already have a credit card–size lock pick set, but some stuff I like to double up on. I always keep a full-size lock pick set in my laptop bag.

Poncho: A poncho is fairly self-explanatory. You can use it if it rains, but you can also use it as an emergency shelter.

QuikClot: I always carry QuikClot in my laptop bag, and have it around anytime I'm teaching a class that involves firearms. QuikClot is basically gauze that's covered in a substance that accelerates the body's natural clotting process. This is something I want to have around if I'm ever shot or stabbed or even if I get a nasty gash in a car accident.

Flashlight: I think it's really important to have a flashlight in an emergency or just a standard power outage. The one I carry is extra small and I call it the Spy Flashlight. You can get a free spy flashlight as a gift from me at SpyFlash light.com.

Multi-tool: I like having a Leatherman multi-tool. It's got a million and one uses thanks to the pliers, knives, screwdrivers, and other tools it has.

Auto jiggler: When we start to talk about escape scenarios, you'll understand why I think an auto jiggler is an important item to have. In the event you need to hotwire or commandeer a car in an emergency, this tool will help you get into an older model car. Remember slugs that could be used in vending machines? An auto jiggler is kind of like a slug key and is basically a lock-picking set for cars. They are used by locksmiths, auto dealers, and towing and repossession companies. You can use it to jiggle open the lock to cars made up until 1999. Also auto jigglers are perfectly legal to carry.

Duct tape: Duct tape has thousands of uses and is a great thing to have around. You can use it to patch a hole in a tent or to attach things together to create a shelter. Duct tape is so sturdy and durable, that there are websites devoted to using it in crazy ways, like making wallets and even a hammock.

Fire source: I don't smoke, but I always carry a lighter. I want to be ready if I ever need to start a fire to keep myself warm or to cook some food.

Paracord: Throughout this book you're going to see how many amazing uses there are for paracord. I keep seven feet of it in my laptop bag. You'll hear a lot more about how I use paracord later on.

Voice recorder: Many phones can record something for you. I still like to carry around a voice recorder. If I'm doing business with someone I don't trust 100 percent, I may go ahead and record the situation. If you want to do this, you need to know what the law says about recording conversations in the state you live in. A one-party state basically means you can record the call, if it's two-party, you have to ask permission. It's easy to find out the law of your particular state online.

Tier Three: Vehicle Gear

Americans spend a lot of time in their cars. Believe it or not, the average American spends four and a third years in their cars and drives enough distance to travel to the moon and back three times. The average American spends a whopping thirty-eight hours a year stuck in traffic. For this reason, it's critical you have some basic survival gear in your car with you at all times. The two items I think you need to have in your car are a toolbox and a seventy-two-hour kit. Both my wife and I have these items in each of our vehicles.

> **Toolbox:** I keep some fairly specific items in the toolbox I keep in my vehicle:
>
> > *Ax:* I keep a small ax in my toolbox. This can come in handy if you need to chop up some wood or cut through a tree blocking a road.
> >
> > *Towrope:* I've actually used this once to haul my cousin's car, which was broken down. A towrope enables you to pull your car out of a tricky situation— and it's also useful in the event you need rope to tie something together, such as securing cargo or making a shelter.
> >
> > *Hand-crank radio:* You don't want to depend on your phone or your car radio for information in an emergency situation. A hand-crank radio enables you to know what's going on at all times (since it's a hand-crank, you don't have to worry about batteries).

Cigarette lighter: You already know I have a lighter in my laptop bag, but to be extra safe, I keep one in my car as well.

Crowbar: A crowbar is useful in the event you need to smash out a window or break through a fence. It can also be used as a pry or a lever.

First-aid kit: I have a simple first-aid kit you can get at most retail stores. You should be able to handle basic injuries and remember to keep QuikClot in there as well.

Local map: If you ever have to leave town in a hurry, you need to be able to navigate local and back roads. You can't depend on your GPS or cell phone in an emergency situation.

Paracord: I like to keep at least twenty feet of paracord in my car at all times. You are probably starting to see that I think paracord is valuable because I have it in my car, in my laptop bag . . . pretty much everywhere.

Knife: I keep a basic survival knife in my car. Yes, I still have one clipped to my pants pocket but it's always a good idea to have more than one knife.

Collapsible shovel: A collapsible shovel is a great thing to have in your car, and I'm a particular fan of the Glock E-tool. It's not unlikely that you'll find yourself in a situation where you just need to dig your tire out of snow or mud. Having this tool makes this fairly easy to do.

Seventy-two-hour kit: A seventy-two-hour kit is an absolutely critical item for you to have in your car. Should you end up in an accident in an obscure area, your car breaks down, or you're trapped in snow, the items in this small backpack can keep you alive. This kit contains three days' worth of food and water. This pack is small; it's not going to take up a lot of space in your car, and it's just not something you can afford to go without. It's easy to buy these packs premade or you can make one yourself. A good pack contains the following items:

Food bars: You want at least six high-energy bars, about four hundred calories each. They should come wrapped in waterproof packaging.

Six boxes of Aqua Blox: This is enough water to last three days. This emergency drinking water is Coast Guard approved and has a five-year shelf life.

Water purification tablets: You should have at least ten purification tablets. Ten tablets will purify as many as five two-liter bottles of water. To use them simply drop them in the water, wait a few minutes, and the water is safe to drink.

AM/FM radio: Make sure you also have batteries. The radio allows you to monitor the weather and other radio stations in the event of an emergency.

LED flashlight: You want a flashlight that is re-chargeable and won't run out of power. Look for a flashlight you can recharge by simply squeezing the handle.

Thirty-hour survival candle: This candle comes with an adjustable wick and can also be used as a small camp stove to heat food.

Five-in-one emergency survival whistle: In addition to the whistle, the five-in-one has a signal mirror, compass, waterproof match container, and flint for starting fires.

Waterproof matches: You want a box of waterproof matches in case your gear gets wet during an emergency.

Emergency sleeping bag: The bag should be waterproof and windproof and retain 90 percent of your body heat.

Emergency poncho: Get a poncho that includes a hood to protect your entire body from the elements.

Survival knife: Some survival knives contain as many as sixteen different tools, including a Phillips-head screwdriver, can opener, corkscrew, reamer, manicure blade, sturdy reamer, hook disgorger, slot-screw driver, key ring, toothpick, fish scaler, tweezers, wood saw, cutting blade, and cap lifter.

Respirator dust mask: You want a mask that is approved by the National Institute for Occupational Safety and Health.

Pocket tissues: Have at least three packs of tissues.

Safety goggles: To protect your eyes from debris during a disaster.

Sewing kit: To use for sewing clothing or to repair tears in tents or other shelters. Make sure you have safety pins, needles, buttons, and thread.

Twenty-four-piece hygiene kit: Consider having a toothbrush, toothpaste, Wetnaps for your hands, a bar of soap, shampoo and conditioner, dental floss pick, hand lotion, body lotion, deodorant, razor, comb, sanitary pads, shaving cream, and a washcloth.

Small first-aid kit: You want to have bandages in different sizes, fabric strips, alcohol pads, and gauze pads.

Deck of playing cards: For entertainment.

Note pad and pencil: For writing down important information during an emergency.

Miscellaneous Items

As you now know, I like to be prepared to deal with anything. In addition to the items I've already gone over in the Three Tiers of Survival Gear, there are a few other things I like to keep in my car. One of these is bolt cutters. If I ever need to cut through a chain link fence, or snap a padlock off of a fence, these are going to work. If you're cutting through fences, you're most likely in an extreme situation. If you haven't figured it out already I also like to double up on certain items. I like to add extra rations of food and water pouches to what's already in my seventy-two-hour kit.

Remember, I'm not saying you need to run out and buy all of these items today. You should think about what items in the Three Tiers of Survival Gear would work best for you. But at the very least, start putting together your survival gear today.

Gathering Intelligence: Collecting Information to Stay Safe

Now that you know which tools you'll need to get through nearly any situation, I'm going to share some essential survival knowledge with you. In addition to preparing yourself for disasters by having food and water and other essentials, there are a few things you should do in advance to keep your family safe.

Sally Gordon was spending Christmas in paradise with her family and friends in luxury villas in Patong, Thailand, back in 2004. Gordon was standing on the beach when she noticed a wave approaching. Not thinking there was anything to worry about, she ran into her villa to grab her camera. In a matter of seconds, a huge wave hit, and the entire villa was ripped away. Gordon was immediately caught up in the powerful current. The water pulled her body through buildings and smashed her against debris, and even pulled her under a floating car. Miraculously, she washed up about a mile inland. She lost several close friends that day in the tsunami that devastated Thailand (as well as India, Sri Lanka, Indonesia, and other countries). She was eventually reunited with her family. One of her sons was able to run about a mile inland and shimmied up a tree, her husband and another son scrambled to the top of the golf clubhouse, and her third son, who was directly hit by the wave, was saved by a fellow tourist who pulled him up a tree. Gordon and her family were incredibly fortunate to survive their ordeal. Of the 250,000 people who died in the tsunami, about 9,000 of them were tourists. Most of the stories about surviving the tsunami start off the same way—"we were in paradise," or we were having a lovely time at the beach. No one could have imagined that such destruction could occur within mere minutes.

HUMINT Abroad: Human Sources Can Save You

Obviously tsunamis are rare, and the tsunami of 2004 was one of the most extreme situations a tourist could encounter. That being said, thousands of tourists were stranded, hurt, and dependent on foreign governments for help while in a country that had just suffered a phenomenal disaster. The CIA uses the term HUMINT (short for human intelligence) to refer to any information that can be gathered from human sources. In other words, this is boots-on-the-ground intelligence gathering. I can't stress enough how important it is to do some basic HUMINT when traveling to a foreign country. Before you leave home, spend some time online studying the country and making sure it's safe enough for you to even visit in the first place. You should talk to people and ask where to find local hospitals, the American embassy, transportation, and escape routes. Should the country you are traveling in be hit with a major disaster like a tsunami, where could you go for medical help? How would you find your family members?

While I'm cautious, I'll admit it's unlikely you'll encounter something as terrible as Sally Gordon did while traveling. However, HUMINT research can simply mean the difference between staying safe and putting yourself at risk. When you're abroad, make a point to note what's typical and what's not. What's the baseline? What are locals wearing? How can you blend in? It's crucial when traveling abroad to not stick out like a sore thumb—you don't want to become a target, and then a victim. In addition to blending like a local, it's a good idea to take note of the following when traveling abroad (or anywhere, really):

> Pay close attention and be sure to follow any travel warnings issued regarding the country you are traveling to.
> Make sure you have the contact information for the nearest U.S. embassy or consulate.
> Note possible exit strategies should you have to flee during a natural disaster or civil unrest.

HUMINT at Home

It's also crucial you take the time to do some reconnaissance in the community where you live. If you've lived in the same place for a long period of time, it becomes very easy to stop paying attention to changes that are happening in your own area. You may remember a time when you're driving with your spouse, and you ask, "Hey, when did that store show up?" You may be surprised when the response is "last year." Whether you've lived in the same place your entire life or you've just moved to a new town, it's essential you gather some intelligence about the place you live. Not too long ago I relocated from Virginia to Utah. One of the first things I did was gather intelligence about my new home. Make sure you know where to find all of the following. In the event of a major disaster, you may need immediate access to some or all of these places:

Exits and chokeholds: If you had to escape on foot or by car, which route would you take? Chokeholds are places where congestion or blockage is likely to occur. If you know where such places exist, you'll be able to avoid them in an emergency.

Hospitals: How far are you from the closest hospital? If that hospital were inaccessible, where would you go?

Pharmacy: It's important to know where you could purchase medications you might need if you or a family member is injured or becomes sick.

Water sources: One of the first things I learned about my new community is that I live about a hundred yards from a river, and about three miles from a lake. Should there be an emergency, I could take one of the water filters I always have, grab a bucket, and gather drinking water for my family. In August 2014, officials in Toledo, Ohio, had to issue a warning to residents that they should not drink their water. The governor declared a state of emergency, and there was a run on bottled water in area stores. You never know when your water supply may be at risk. Knowing where you can access water is critical for your family's survival in an emergency situation.

The police department: Always know the exact location of your closest police department. This is where you would need to drive if someone was following you in a vehicle or you're faced with any sort of emergency.

Your local municipal airport: I highly recommend that everyone learn the location of your municipal airport. I paid a visit to mine when I moved to Utah. And for about $100, I was able to take a "discovery flight." The discovery flight helps you see where you'd go if there was a serious emergency. It's helpful to know where the hangar is and where the planes are stored. Most municipal airports also offer cool stuff like flight clubs and flying lessons. But the real reason you need to know about your municipal airport? In an extreme situation—I'm talking end-of-the-world style disaster—a municipal airport is going to give you your best chance at getting out of Dodge. In this situation you'd either pay someone (another reason to keep cash around), or hope someone would take pity on you and help you out. For this reason, it's not a bad idea to get to know a pilot or two.

Food and Water: Build Your Supply

I recommend keeping up to a year's supply of food and water for yourself and your family. Not only will this keep you alive in an emergency but it will give you peace of mind knowing that if you suffer a job loss, you'll be able to feed your family. Obviously not everyone will have the financial resources (or storage space) to keep this much, but the more you can keep, the better.

Steps You Must Take Immediately If a Crisis Occurs

In the event there is a major disaster—whether it's a natural disaster, a riot, or any type of catastrophic occurrence—you must do whatever it takes to get out of the dangerous situation.

1. Remember, movement saves lives, so *get off the X*. Moving and taking action significantly increases your chances of survival. It's those who don't move who are going to be killed.

2. Quickly arm yourself. Ideally you'll have had a chance to arm yourself with your knife or gun (at the very least I'm hoping your tactical pen was on you), but if the need arises, almost anything can be a weapon, including a rock, a shard of broken glass, or even a big stick.

3. Get your gear if you can safely do so. Obviously having access to your seventy-two-hour kit is preferable. If you are able to get it, do so. If it's putting you in greater danger to get it, you will have to leave it behind.

Water

The recommended amount of water to have on hand is one gallon per person per day. Some people like to use fifty-five-gallon containers. I happen to like the seven-gallon reliance aquatainer. Obviously a gallon per person per day adds up quickly.

How Much Cash Do You Recommend a Person Keep in the House for Emergencies?

While some is better than none, I would make it your goal to keep at least $1,000 in cash, in twenties, in your home at all times. I'd keep more than that if you can. This will cover you for a while should some emergency arise that prevents you from getting access to cash from the bank. It will give you peace of mind to know that you can use cash to pay people to help you and your family escape in a crisis—or buy something you may need after a natural disaster or blackout.

Food Storage

I realize most of us can't go out and buy a year's supply of food all at once. You can start to collect canned food and grains each month, and before you know it you'll have a year's supply of food (or whatever quantity works for you). I happen to be a member of the Church of Jesus Christ of Latter-Day Saints (Mormon), and I get my food from an LDS cannery. Anyone of any religion can buy food from the cannery, and they have the best prices around. There are currently 101 canneries where you can purchase items in bulk. If you can't get to a cannery, you can purchase food online at ProvidentLiving.org. Again, remember that you do not have to be Mormon to purchase food at one of the canneries. They are open to everyone regardless of religious affiliation.

4

BECOME AN ESCAPE ARTIST

How to Easily Escape Rope, Handcuffs, Zip Ties, and Duct Tape

A woman was in the office at the tanning salon where she worked when she noticed a man on the surveillance camera. She was the only employee in the salon at the time. All of a sudden, the man was standing at the door to her office. She was struck over the head and pulled into a van, where her legs and wrists were duct taped together. Luckily, this woman managed to escape by throwing herself out of the van. She suffered a fractured skull and other injuries, but could have suffered a much darker fate. Turns out, forty-nine-year-old Kelly Swoboda had basically transformed his van into a moveable torture chamber—by outfitting it with chains that were mounted to the floor as well as zip ties and ropes. Swoboda was discovered to have notes on about twenty different women. He was following them around and had noted their license plate numbers.

Most of us have duct tape lying around the house. We use it for packing up boxes or repairing something that needs a quick fix.

However, most people don't know that duct tape has a much more sinister use. If a criminal wants to restrain you during a kidnapping or home invasion, they are most likely going to do so with duct tape. The fact is, once a criminal wraps duct tape around a victim's wrist, most people mentally give up because they have no idea how to escape from it. However, I know how to break out of it in just a couple of seconds and by the end of this chapter so will you. You'll also know how to break out of zip ties and escape from handcuffs from the trunk of a car. I have successfully taught these techniques to men and women of all ages (ages nine to seventy-seven, to be exact) from many different backgrounds. My students have found that knowing how to break out of restraints in an emergency situation is empowering and instills confidence.

How to Escape Duct Tape

A Criminal's Favorite Restraint

Kelly Swoboda is by no means the first criminal to use duct tape. It's the easiest and fastest way to restrain someone. Once you see how easy it can be to get out of, you'll never be intimidated by it again. I'm not a huge, threatening guy, but because I know what to do, I can get out of duct tape in seconds. I've had the opportunity to work with mixed martial artists—huge guys with massive arms. I've taped their wrists and asked them to escape. These seriously strong guys will try to pry their hands apart, pulling and pulling on the tape, and they get no results. Being duct taped is psychologically draining. If you don't know how to get out of it, and you're just pulling at the tape, you're eventually going to give up.

The key to breaking out of duct tape isn't strength, but knowing how to re-create the angle that makes it easy to rip. If you've ever torn off a piece of tape (which I'm sure you have) then you know that if you want to rip the tape you simply tear it at the correct angle. That's basically what we're going to do here.

Step 1: Positioning

When you are being duct taped, lean forward as far as you can, pressing your elbows and forearms closely together. If you are able to, make fists with your hands. The idea here is to create a tight seal with your forearms. Leaning forward also puts you in the "submissive position," which signals to your attackers that you're not going to be a problem.

Step 2: The Break

Remember, you can pull as hard as you want to, and that tape isn't going to break. You need to re-create an angle that will easily tear the tape. To do this, raise your arms as high above your head as possible. In one quick, swift motion, pull your arms *down and out to the sides* as if you're quickly pulling your hands past each hip. You can watch a free video of me doing this duct tape escape at SpySecretsBook.com.

Troubleshooting

While you're practicing, if you find the tape isn't breaking right away, it's most likely because you are not pulling your arms and hands apart to the side past your hips. Practice the maneuver until you have mastered the movement—a quick, sharp down and apart motion that starts above your head, and ends with you pulling your hands to the side past your hips. The tape will tear once you've successfully mastered this motion.

Plan B: If You Are Taped from Behind or Injured

I'm often asked what happens if a criminal tapes your hands behind you. Chances are, this isn't going to happen, and a criminal is going to tape your hands in front of you because it's faster and easier. Plus it allows them to grab your hands so they can lead you where they want to take you. However, should this happen—or should you have sustained an injury that prevents you from re-creating the angle necessary to break the tape, I'm going to teach you a second escape method. While this method is different, the goal remains the same, to re-create the angle that breaks the tape. The alternative method requires

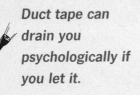

Duct tape can drain you psychologically if you let it.

that you find something that has a ninety-degree angle—the corner of a wall, a chair, a piece of furniture—anything, and simply put your taped hands in the middle of the edge and do a sawing motion until it tears. If you decide to practice this method as well, you'll be surprised how quickly the tape will break open.

How to Escape from Zip Ties

While duct tape remains the most common method criminals use to restrain someone, it is also important that you know how to

Your Hands, Feet, and Mouth
Are Covered in Duct Tape. What Would You Do?

I would free my hands first. This is always the first priority and I would do it exactly as I taught you earlier in this chapter. Next, I would lift the tape off of my mouth so I could breathe better. Last, I would tear the tape off of my feet and legs.

It's important to remember that duct tape can drain you psychologically if you let it. If you're covered in duct tape it's easy to give up. Don't. The fact is, a seventeen-year-old girl who took my class with her dad actually wanted to give this a try being fully "duct taped up." She voluntarily let us cover her practically head to toe in tape. Her legs were taped to about six inches up past her knees, and her arms were covered to the elbows. We also put tape on her mouth. This girl got herself completely free from all of the tape in less than thirty seconds. Not allowing yourself to be intimidated by the tape is just as important as knowing the technique to get out of it.

escape from zip ties should you ever need to. In Jacksonville, Florida, two women, ages eighteen and nineteen, were found dead on the side of the road. Both of the bodies were bound with zip ties. In Chico, California, a physician's assistant was pulled over for a traffic violation. Turns out, he had a history of kidnapping college-aged women, and then sexually assaulting them. The women had their hands and feet bound with zip ties, and tape covering their eyes.

Like duct tape, zip ties are difficult to break out of, if you don't know the correct technique. They are cheap, accessible, and like duct tape, zip ties are psychologically taxing—it's easy for a victim to believe he won't be able to escape.

Step 1: Positioning

While being zip tied, you will want to put your arms out as far in front of you as possible, with your forearms held tightly together. This is the same positioning you used for escaping from duct tape.

Step 2: Rotate the Lock

You will see that the zip tie holding your hands together has a small lock. You must rotate that lock so that it is placed directly where the palms of your hands meet. It doesn't need to be perfect, but get it as close to the center as possible. Since you obviously won't be able to use your hands to do this, you'll need to bite the end of the zip tie with your teeth, and rotate the lock into the correct position.

Step 3: The Break

The technique for breaking zip ties is exactly the same as it is with duct tape. You want to raise your hands as high above your head as possible, keeping your forearms tightly together. In one swift movement, you will pull your arms directly down and to the side past your hips. The lock will pop open. You can watch a video of me escaping from zip ties at SpySecretsBook.com.

Swap Your Shoelaces

If you don't want to carry paracord in your briefcase or purse, consider swapping out your normal shoelaces for paracord laces. They are easy to find, come in many different colors, and don't look any different from regular laces.

Troubleshooting

Escaping zip ties using this method takes a lot more strength and not everyone can do it. You have to get the perfect angle of pulling your arms and hands apart as you come down. If the angle isn't perfect it's not going to work. If you can't get out this way, don't worry, because there's a second method.

Plan B: The Paracord Method

While it's been my experience that anyone can escape from duct tape using the break method, as I just mentioned, zip ties can be more difficult for some people. Fortunately there is an alternative method. Remember the paracord I talked about in the previous chapter? This is where it's going to come in handy.

Take your paracord out of your pocket, bag, or shoes. Ideally, you need about seven feet of paracord. Insert the paracord through the zip tie so that it's hanging down in the center of your hands. Next, tie a loop on each end that is large enough for you to put your foot in. Place your feet into the loops of paracord, and recline on your back. Make a bicycling motion with your feet braced in the loops, and you will literally saw right through the zip tie.

How to Escape from Rope

Eleven days after a married couple went missing from New Orleans, their bodies were found in the Intracoastal Waterway. Their feet were bound with blue nylon rope. The man's rope was tethered to a thirty-pound kettlebell. The rope around the woman's feet was frayed, which suggests it had also been attached to something. Leonila Tara Cortez left in a car with a male friend on August 21, 1996, and was never seen alive again. Her family knew something was wrong, as she would never leave behind her two young children. While it took years to correctly identify her body, it was clear that her body had been bound with rope. Again, rope isn't used as commonly as duct tape, but it's critical you know how to get out of rope should you find yourself in an extreme situation.

Step 1: The Position

When you are being tied up, you want to keep your palms together, but your elbows need to be apart. You *do not* want to press your forearms together the way you would if you were being duct taped. The idea here is to create extra space from the curve in your wrists when you keep your elbows apart.

Step 2: Forward and Shimmy

After you've been tied up while keeping your elbows apart, move your arms forward until they are completely straight and also make sure your hands are flat and pressed together. Once you have done this, begin to shimmy your hands back and forth quickly and eventually you'll be able to pull one of your hands free. This technique will work regardless of the thickness of the rope, but know that if the rope is thinner, it will take more time and you'll likely get rope burn. If you want to see exactly how to do this, I've created a video for you at SpySecretsBook.com.

Plan B: Escaping Rope with Paracord

Hopefully you're starting to see why it's such a good idea to keep paracord around—or to at least swap out your regular shoelaces for paracord laces. This method is a good backup in case the criminal you encountered is great at tying knots. This technique takes more time—from thirty seconds to five minutes, so you'd want to use this method if you've been tossed in a room alone. You will craft two loops onto each end of a long piece of paracord, and insert the paracord through center of the rope between your hands (just as you did when escaping zip ties). You'll have a loop falling down on each side of the rope. Insert your feet into the loops, recline backward and do the bicycling motion with your feet until you saw straight through the rope.

How to Escape from Handcuffs

Handcuffs, as you know by now, are not a criminal's preferred method of restraining a person, but it's a good idea to know how to break out of them anyway. You'll be amazed by how easy it is to do this. All you really need is a couple of cheap items. You may already have these things lying around the house—a bobby pin or a barrette.

Method 1: The Bobby Pin

This is why I always carry a bobby pin. You can easily turn an inexpensive, everyday bobby pin into a tool that will open handcuffs in seconds. If you're traveling overseas, I highly recommend you keep this tool in your pocket, already made.

Step 1: The Tool

A set of pliers will make bending the bobby pin exactly the way we need it much easier. Simply use the pliers to straighten out the bobby pin into one straight line. One side of the bobby pin is smooth, and the other has ridges. Take off the little nub on the end of the smooth side of the bobby pin. (You can take it off by clamping down on it with your pliers and stripping it off.) You want to make a minuscule upward bend on the end of the smooth side of the bobby pin. I'm talking about maybe a quarter inch, at about a forty-five-degree angle. You're basically making a tiny shovel.

Step 2: Escape the Cuffs

For the purposes of these instructions, I'm talking about using your right hand. Hold your hand so that the teeth of the cuffs (the part that goes into the handcuffs) is on the bottom. You only need to be concerned with the keyhole of the handcuff. The keyhole is a small circle that has a small slot shooting off of the right side. You want to insert your shovel into the small slot portion of the keyhole (you don't want to be in the round portion at all, just the small slot) and insert the bobby pin into that small slot until you feel it hitting metal. As soon as it hits metal, you pull the bobby pin down toward the ground and then to the right. It's important to note these are two distinct motions. Once the bobby pin is inserted, you first pull down and then you pull to the side . . . don't try pulling at an angle or the cuffs won't open.

Troubleshooting

- For the purposes of practicing, know that it's entirely possible that you'll take the small bend out of your bobby pin. Simply bend the end back upward into that minuscule angle and try again.
- Make sure you are pulling down and to the right and that you are smooth and gentle. This is not a process that requires a lot of force at all.

Method 2: A Shim Made from a Barrette

Step 1: The Tool

You'll need a simple basic hair barrette, a hair clip that snaps closed. Again, this is a tool you'll want to make in advance. Your ultimate goal is to turn the barrette into a shim that can be used to block the teeth of the handcuffs so they don't click shut. The first thing you'll need to do is break off the middle piece. You can just bend it upward and snap it off. Then you'll want to break off the fatter, round portion on the top. You can use your pliers to bend this section back and forth until it pops off. Now you have two thinner pieces of metal attached at one end that form a V. The ends of your V will likely be curved upward, so take your pliers and straighten them out. You want the ends of the hair barrette to be as straight as possible.

Step 2: Insert the Shim

For this method, you're only going to be working with the part of the handcuffs where the teeth are inserted into the cuff. You're going to take your barrette that you turned into a shim, and insert it into the space where the teeth go into the cuff. You're going to have to push down on the teeth of the cuffs and then immediately push the shim all the way down. Pushing on the teeth first gives you momentum to push the shim down. Once you've pushed the shim all the way down until it can't go anymore, you will simply hold it in place and then lift your hand out of the cuffs. (The shim blocks the teeth of the cuffs so it won't stay closed and you can open it.) Go to SpySecretsBook.com to watch a video demonstrating how to escape from handcuffs using both a bobby pin and a hair barrette.

A Note on the Trunk Challenge

One of the most challenging and exciting exercises I teach in my Spy Escape and Evasion course is the Trunk Challenge. After mastering the art of getting out of handcuffs, students take their new skills to another level. We take turns practicing escaping from a locked trunk, handcuffed, with a hood over our heads. It sounds like it would be hard, but because my students know exactly what to do, they make it out, sometimes in mere seconds, with the vast majority of people escaping in less than two minutes.

If you want to be adventurous and re-create the trunk challenge that we do in my course, there are a couple of things you should know. First, take your time and go slowly. The trunk of a car is a small, confined space, your blood pressure is going to go up and you're going to feel compelled to move faster. Don't. Take your time and move slowly. If you drop your bobby pin or shim, it's going to be really hard to find it in the dark. Also know that all newer cars have a glow-in-the-dark emergency release pull. You should be able to locate that without too much trouble. What if you're in an older model car that doesn't have an emergency release? Should this ever happen to you, don't panic. Trunk locks are not especially strong. Get on all fours, and push against the trunk with your back—it will hopefully pop open, depending on the vehicle model. Other options? Kick out the backseat. If you're going to attempt this challenge, be sure to practice the above-described escape methods first—and have a friend with you to let you out if you run into any problems.

You've Been Kidnapped—Now What?

You should do absolutely everything in your power to fight off a potential kidnapper. This is not a time to be compliant, but to kick, hit, scream, and use a weapon. Jessica Garner of Redding, California, was walking down the street when a man made a motion to her suggesting she look at items he was selling out of his Ford Explorer. When Garner walked away, the man grabbed her shirt and began to drag her toward his vehicle. She kicked at the man and was able to break free. The man drove off. A quick-thinking teenager who had been kidnapped and forced to drive a woman from New Jersey to Philadelphia purposely crashed into a police officer's car. The teen was able to tell the officer what happened and the kidnapper was arrested on the spot. Not everyone is as lucky. Carlesha Freeland-Gaither was abducted while walking home from a party for her godson. Surveillance video footage shows a man pulling his car over to the side of the road, approaching Freeland-Gaither, and dragging her down the street. At one point she manages to pull her attacker away from the car, but ultimately, she is forced inside.

If you are not able to fight off kidnappers, you need to know that the first twenty-four hours are critical. This is one of the few things they get right in the movies. Once kidnappers have you in their possession, they're likely to move you around. It's possible they'll move you to a safe house, or even move you several times, making it more difficult for you to be found. Whatever you need to do, make sure you escape within those first twenty-four hours. Besides getting moved to a faraway location, you're likely at your strongest during this part of the ordeal. In other words, you've probably got a belly full of food and plenty of water in you. However, three weeks from now you'll probably be a lot weaker and it will be much tougher for you to escape because your captors aren't likely to feed you well and you won't be able to keep up your strength.

Once it's become clear you cannot fight off your attackers, you'll need to put on an act of compliance. Do not look directly at your kidnapper, and be submissive. However, just because you're acting compliant and timid doesn't mean you are giving up—it's all an act. The reason you want to act submissive is that you do not want the kidnappers to think you require additional security measures. If they've duct taped you, and you're screaming your head off, you don't want them to decide to padlock you in the trunk because you're being a problem. While you're acting compliant, you want to be thinking as carefully as you can about how to escape. You're looking for that quick lapse in security that will enable you to break free. So, as soon as you see an opening to escape and your captors aren't around, make a run for it.

Your Inner Spy: Picking Locks, Leaping over Fences and Hot-Wiring Cars

I don't recommend jumping over barbed wire fences just for practice—but in the event you're ever in a real escape and evasion situation, it's good to know how to do this. And I'm certainly not going to suggest you ever hot-wire a car, since that would be illegal (unless it's your own car—and you don't want to do that either, since it will seriously damage the car). I do advocate knowing how to do it, so you're prepared if hot-wiring a car and driving away is the only thing that will save your life.

The Barbed Wire Fence

What you'll need: A heavy flat material that can be used to cover the barbed wire while you're scaling over the fence. A thick blanket, a mattress, or very large pieces of cardboard in a pinch.

How it works: While you would want to be extremely careful going over a barbed wire fence, it's not that difficult to do. You'll take whatever material you have found to cover the barbed wire fence, toss it over the fence, and cross the fence at that section.

The Razor Wire Fence

A razor wire fence is designed to seriously cut you. If you try to climb over a razor wire fence there is a good chance you will be cut so badly that you will bleed out and die—or at least not make it very far. At a portion of the Mexican border, a man was recently trapped in the razor wire trying to cross into the United States. It took emergency crews almost an hour to cut him out. In one year alone, twenty-one people had to be rescued from the razor wire. This is something you only want to do if absolutely necessary, and you'll want to use extreme caution.

What you'll need: A team of people, a cane or other type of curved stick, a flat material such as you would use for climbing over a barbed wire fence.

How it works: Two people on the team will take the cane or other long object and hook it onto the razor wire and pull the loops of razor wire down until they are flat. While two members of the team are holding the razor wire flat, the others will cover the razor wire with the flat surface and climb over. Once the first set of team members has crossed the fence, they will use the cane or long object to hold the fence flat while the remaining members cross.

How to Hot-Wire a Car

I seriously hope that none of us ever ends up in a situation so chaotic and desperate that your only choice is to hot-wire a car to escape. Before we go any further, there's one thing I need to be clear about. *You cannot practice this technique on your car—or anyone else's for that matter.* This will do serious damage to the car. I do know one person who actually found himself in a situation where he needed to use this method. He was swimming, in a swimming hole in the middle of nowhere. Guess what? He left his car keys in his shorts and lost his keys in the swimming hole. Luckily, his car was an older model vehicle, and he had tools in his car. He was able to follow these instructions, hot-wire his car, and get himself home. Obviously this guy was in a tough spot, but don't forget that doing this will really mess up your car.

The Right Car

Before we get into the specifics, I want to take a moment to talk about procuring a car to hot-wire in a dire emergency. First, take a look around and see if there are any cars with unlocked doors, or keys just sitting there in the seat. The real jackpot would be finding an unlocked tow truck. Why? Tow trucks have a master set of keys, and this set is basically going to get you into any car around. Obviously a tow truck might not be right there for the taking, or you won't find a car that's unlocked. Your next best bet is to find an older model car—I'm talking 1999 and before.

These older model cars are actually everywhere. Once people start noticing them, they are often surprised that there are so many older model cars still out there. Make a point of looking for them when you're out on the road. I guarantee you'll start seeing them everywhere.

What You'll Need
- Wire cutters and strippers
- Pliers
- Flathead and Phillips-head screwdrivers
- Hammer
- Insulated gloves
- A car
- Electrical tape

How it works: This is a rather simple process, but I'd recommend keeping a set of these instructions in your car, or maybe your laptop bag or purse, for a dire emergency. Since this isn't a technique you can practice, it's entirely possible you won't remember how to do it in an emergency situation.

1. Once you've found the car you're going to hot-wire, insert a flathead screwdriver into the ignition as you would a key. Pound the screwdriver into the ignition with your hammer. You will want to turn the screwdriver just as you would a key that's in the ignition. If you're having trouble turning the screwdriver, use your pliers to help you. Sometimes, if you're really lucky, this action is enough to start the car.
2. Use a Phillips-head screwdriver to remove the screws in the plastic panel above and below your steering column. When the panels are removed you're going to see several wires under the steering column.

Breaking Car Windows

Should you ever need to break into a car to save your life, and you need to do this undetected, duct tape is going to be very helpful. Place large pieces of tape on the window in an X. This will keep the glass from shattering everywhere and making noise. Also, to break the window, use your tactical pen, or another object, to strike the window at the corners. This is where the glass is tightest and most likely to break. If you strike the window in the center, and the object is not strong enough, it's just going to bounce off.

3. Locate the two red wires. These wires provide power to the vehicle.
4. Put on your insulated gloves.
5. Cut both ends of the red wires and strip the ends. Twist the ends of the two red wires together. (One red wire from each of the wires you cut. So don't twist the ends of the same wire, but the two different wires together.)
6. Locate the brown wires; these wires connect to the starter. Some cars will have one brown wire, others will have two.
7. Cut both of the brown wires and strip the ends.
8. **If there are two brown wires:** Touch the two brown wires together to start the car. *Once the car is started, do not let the wires touch again. They must be kept separate.* You can wrap them with electrical tape to keep them

from touching. This will also keep you from getting shocked.

If there is one brown wire: If the car has only one brown wire, touch the brown wire to the red wires to start the car. Once the car starts, separate the wires, and put electrical tape over the end of the one brown wire.

Picking Locks

It should absolutely go without saying that you shouldn't pick anyone's lock . . . unless they ask you to. In fact, I'm asked to do it all the time in my neighborhood. If anyone gets locked out, I'm the guy they go to. Lock pick sets are inexpensive and fun to use, and if you follow these instructions, you'll be the person the neighbors call when they've lost their keys. Before we go on, you can see the credit card–size lock pick set that I use at SafeHomeGear.com. Also, because I'm often asked, you won't damage a lock if you practice picking it five or ten times. However, if you do it hundreds of times you will damage a lock. In other words, picking the lock on your front door every now and then won't do it any harm. But if you spend two hours a day practicing on the lock then you'll need to replace it.

How Safe Is Your Lock?

Before we get into actual lock picking, I want to talk about how important it is that you have a good safe lock on your home. I was in the Salt Lake area not too long ago when I decided to pop into my brother's new house. He wasn't home, but that wasn't a problem. Within a few seconds I was inside his house and helping myself to his snacks. My brother, like most Americans, had an incredibly easy lock to pick. About 75 percent of locks on doors are made by Kwikset, and in my experience they are incredibly easy to open with simple tools. A common criminal is not likely to have a problem picking your lock if you have a Kwikset lock. These locks are used by contractors everywhere because they are easy to come by (you can get them at any big-box building supply store), and of course, inexpensive. I highly recommend you replace your locks if you have Kwikset. It's not a huge investment, and your family will be safer as a result. Schlage and Medeco are two brands of locks that I personally like to use.

The L Rake and the Tension Wrench

All you need to pick a lock are an L rake and a tension wrench. I carry both of these around with me at all times in my credit card lock pick set. The hardest part about picking a lock is finding the correct amount of pressure when you use the tension wrench. If you use too much tension, the lock is going to think it's some kind of intrusion and not open. You're using a minimal amount of tension. Basically you need to dial back whatever you think is right about ten times. So remember this when you're inserting the tension wrench in the following step. Also be aware that lock picking takes finesse. The more you practice, the faster you'll be able to determine if you're executing the technique properly.

Step 1: Insert the Tension Wrench

Again, using a featherweight pressure, insert the tension wrench into the bottom of the lock. The long portion of the tool will be hanging off to the side. Place your finger on the tension wrench and apply an absolutely minimal amount of pressure.

Step 2: Insert the L Rake

Note: You must keep consistent pressure on the tension wrench the entire time you are picking the lock. If you apply additional pressure, it's not going to work.

You're going to insert the L rake into the lock with the ridged portion on top. You're going to scrape the L rake back and forth while applying slight pressure toward the top of the L rake. Think of the L rake as a toothbrush and you're brushing the teeth of the lock . . . that's the motion you want to use going in and out of the lock.

Step 3: Locate the Fifth Pin

Note: You've successfully picked a lock when you've tricked the lock into believing all five pins have been have been manipulated properly. It's really common to have four pins moved after just a few seconds, and then you'll need to change your movement to locate that fifth pin.

To locate the fifth pin, you're going to change the movement you're making with the L rake. You are now going to jerk the L rake up and down, making sure you're still going all the way to the front and the back of the lock. When the fifth pin is hit, you feel pressure on the tension wrench, and the lock will open.

Some people in my course get this down right away, while it takes longer for others. Lock picking, while not hard to do, takes practice. Once you get the feel of how to manipulate the tools in a way that hits all the pins, you'll be able to pick a lock within seconds. Also the beauty of this technique is that not only can you use this to open door locks, but also padlocks and even filing cabinets. (Rachael Ray had me on her show and I demonstrated how to pick a filing cabinet lock in less than thirty seconds. To watch a video where I show you how to pick locks, visit SpySecretsBook.com.)

5

THE IMPENETRABLE HOME

How to Criminal Proof Your House

It was around 3 a.m. when I heard the noise. It was loud enough that it woke up my wife as well. None of our alarms had gone off— but I knew I had to immediately determine whether someone had gotten into our home. I launched into my simple but well-practiced home defense plan. I grabbed my flashlight off of my nightstand, opened my safe, grabbed my gun, and went to the top of the stairs. I did all of this in less than seven seconds.

After not hearing any noise and making an announcement to get out of my house, I went downstairs to clear the house. It turned out there wasn't an intruder at all. An air mattress had crashed down from a shelf, making a loud thud. Everything was fine that night at my house—but unfortunately many Americans aren't as lucky as my family was.

Home invasions can happen anywhere to anyone. In Millburn, New Jersey, a suburb of New York City, a man burst into a home where he violently beat a mother of two for ten minutes. The attack was captured on film thanks to a nanny cam. It turns out that the suspect had a violent past, with twelve prior criminal convictions. In Staten Island, New York, sixty-seven-year-old Peter Gialluisi unknowingly walked in on a burglar in his garage after returning home from a family party. He was fatally stabbed, and his wife was seriously injured.

Home invasions are on the rise. Many people think, "That won't happen to me" when they hear a news story about a home invasion. But there are a few statistics from the FBI that you should be aware of:

- One in five homes will be the victim of a break-in or home invasion.
- 85% of burglars case homes before a home invasion.
- 50% of burglars portray service men (FedEx, UPS, etc.) before a home invasion.
- 94% of burglars are high on drugs when they are invading a home.
- 30% of violent assaults take place during a home invasion.
- 60% of rapes take place during a home invasion.
- 33% of burglars enter the home through an unopened door or window.

There are also two kinds of burglars. Your day burglar is a professional. This is the guy who will have already cased your house. He knows when you're away, and he's going to break in when you're at work. You will have no idea that he was there until your go to look for your diamond bracelet or your laptop computer. While I certainly hope you don't encounter a daytime burglar, you should know that nighttime burglars are an even greater concern. This is because the guy who is going to rob you in the middle of the night is dangerous. This guy is most likely high on drugs or mentally ill, and he doesn't care whether you're home or not. In fact, he may want you to be home. If you're home, you can tell him where you keep the extra cash or how to get in the safe. These guys are ruthless, and you don't want them anywhere near you or your family.

Think Like a Criminal

While all of this might sound incredibly scary, there is some good news. By putting ourselves in the mind-set of a criminal, we can easily determine whether our homes are appealing to them. Some very simple, inexpensive changes can help a criminal decide that he wants to skip your house altogether.

Tactic One: Case Your Own Neighborhood

How a Nice Family Walk Can Prevent a Break-In

The first strategy is literally as easy as taking a stroll down your street, but what you learn on this walk may stop a burglar from breaking into your house. What do you see when you look at all the other houses on your block? Put yourself in the mind-set of a burglar. Which house would you want to rob? Which houses looks inhabited—like someone is home right now? Which houses give away signals that someone hasn't been around? Look for the signals that a burglar seeks out to determine whether someone is home. Observe newspapers, mail, or any other papers that are delivered. Are newspapers lying in a pile on the sidewalk? Is mail bursting out of the mailbox? What do the lawns look like? Are they mowed and well cared for? Who leaves their garage door open (more on that in a bit)? These are all open invitations to burglars—they all suggest that the house is unoccupied. It's also especially important to bring in the trash cans after the garbage is picked up. It's easy for burglars to figure out when trash day is, and then note who still has their trash cans out a few days later, meaning that homeowner is probably out of town. You want your home to project a secure image. Noting who has these particular items in check is the first step toward making sure your house appears to be the most secure house on the street.

Are You Expecting a Package?

In a quiet New York City neighborhood, a thirty-four-year-old man answered the door for a man with a FedEx package. The individual was hit in the face with a gun when he opened the door, and robbed by three armed men. A couple of thousand dollars in cash, an iPhone and jewelry were taken. In Bowie, Maryland, Richard Peeks was doing yard work at his home when he was approached by a man dressed as a FedEx employee carrying a box. The "FedEx worker" asked Peeks for a glass of water, and before he knew what was happening, the guy pulled out a gun. A St. Louis, Missouri, woman is lucky to be alive after a confrontation with a fake UPS driver. A man posed as a UPS delivery person and told Bernice Cook that he had a package for her. He was holding a cardboard box and a clipboard. He forced his way into her home and proceeded to bind her hands and wrists with duct tape. He then duct taped her to the handle of her kitchen stove and demanded money and jewelry.

It's crucial to be cautious when accepting packages. If you're not expecting something, don't answer the door. If you want to confirm whether a delivery person is real, locate the number to the company yourself and call to confirm if there is a package for you. Obviously, if you feel threatened you should call the police immediately . . . but don't simply believe someone just because he shows up in a uniform and claims to work for a particular company.

If you're not expecting something, don't answer the door.

It's Not Just the Delivery Man You Need to Be Concerned About

Many of us have come home to find a sticker from UPS or FedEx indicating there's a package for us. The next time this happens, remove the sticker immediately, and make sure there really is a package. Be on the lookout for anything stuck to your doors and windows in general. Peter Hart of Fresh Meadows, Queens, was lucky that he noticed a piece of black electrical tape on his window. He told CBS New York, "The first initial thought was, what the heck is it?" Then he realized, "Could that be someone that's marking the house?" Tape, like FedEx slips, can be used by burglars to mark a house they've been casing. If the tape is still there a few days later, they'll assume the person isn't home and will proceed with their plans to break in. In Ireland, criminal gangs took this practice to a new level. Chalk markings started appearing outside of homes in Dublin and Limerick. Turns out, the symbols are used by a recon unit to communicate information to burglars. They used a variety of symbols that conveyed "good target," "too risky," "nothing worth stealing," "wealthy," "alarmed house," "already been burgled," and the even more disturbing "nervous and afraid" and "vulnerable female easily conned." Being aware of any papers, flyers, or unusual markings on your home is essential for keeping you and your family safe.

Tactic Two: Case Your Own House

Most of us probably spend more time than we'd like to taking care of our homes. We want our houses to look inviting and attractive. We mow our lawns, plant flowers, and take pride in our landscaping. However, it's entirely possible we're attracting more than we bargained for with our hard work. Criminals are looking at our houses too—carefully calculating how easy it would be to break in and help themselves to our valuables. Unfortunately, some of the things we may be doing to make our houses look more desirable are telling criminals to come on in and help themselves. That's why it's important to not only case your neighborhood but to case your house, just like a criminal would, to see what elements of your home are making you vulnerable to criminal activity.

Walk around the entire perimeter of your home. Note any places where a criminal could potentially hide, including any overgrown shrubs or bushes. You want to make sure that if someone is in your yard, either you or your neighbors are easily going to see them.

Also look for symbols that suggest your home is full of valuables. Is there an expensive car parked in your driveway? Is your extremely large flat screen TV easily visible from the front yard because you forgot to close the blinds? I'm not suggesting that you make your house look shabby, or that you don't enjoy your fancy car if you have one. That being said, you want to be careful about advertising your valuables to potential criminals. The less they know about what you have, the better.

Clean Up for Safety

While a child's scooter or bicycle in the front yard might seem completely innocent, it's important that these items are always carefully stored away and locked up at the end of the day. A scooter makes an excellent device for breaking glass windows. The same goes for any tools or other objects that can be used as a projectile. Any garden implements, shovels, or other tools need to be out of sight and securely locked.

Tactic Three: Case Your House at Night

While you can learn a lot by casing your house during the day, it's important to repeat the process at night. Walk the perimeter and think about where you'd hide if you were a criminal. Would you know if there was someone hiding behind the area where you keep your trashcans? Is it too dark to tell? Note dark spots where criminals could hide, especially near your front door. Pay attention to lighting. Is the perimeter of your home well lit? Would you be able to see an intruder approaching? Take note of what the weaknesses are. I'll address these issues in a moment when we talk about physical and psychological tricks that will keep criminals away.

Don't Forget About the Garage

A violent robbery in Indianapolis could have been prevented if the garage door had been locked. At approximately 7:30 a.m., four men forced their way into a home, threatening a man, his wife, and his daughter. They took cell phones, cash, and car keys. The incident turned violent, and the woman was shot in the leg. Turns out, the family had forgotten to shut their garage door, providing an easy entrance point for the criminals. Make a point of locking the door in your house that leads to the garage, just as you would your front door.

It's easy to forget to close the garage door itself. We're opening it to get out bikes and scooters for kids or maybe we're hauling out garbage to the curb. We forget that for most of us, access to the garage means access to the house. It's also important to block site lines into the garage. You don't want criminals knowing if there are valuables in the garage, or seeing whether or not there's a car inside. No car usually means no one is home.

You also need to find a safe storage place for your garage door opener. I know it's convenient to leave it in your car, but think twice about keeping it there when you're not in your car. Criminals know that most people leave their garage door openers in their cars. If they want to gain access to your home, all they have to do is break open your car window and grab the garage door opener. To ensure you won't hear them doing this, they'll simply put duct tape on your car window to minimize the sound of the glass breaking. Last, if you're going away for an extended period of time, padlock your garage. Obviously this isn't something you want to be bothered with every day, but it's an extra security measure worth taking if you're on vacation.

Psychological and Physical Tricks

In addition to physical security such as motion-detector lights, deadbolts, and an alarm system, it is possible to secure your home using a powerful combination of physical and psychological tricks. These tricks are easy and inexpensive and will make burglars think twice about robbing your home.

Home Security Signage

As I've said, it's great to have an actual security system, but whether you have one or not, the signs alone are a big deterrent. This may sound silly, but if a burglar thinks there is even a chance you have an alarm system, they will likely move on to the next house that has no signs at all. This is why you need a sign for your yard. Security signs are usually about two feet high and on a pole. Place the sign in a prominent spot in your front yard. You'll also want to put the security stickers in as many windows as possible. I'd recommend placing them on any windows near doorways, as well as basement windows. Sliding glass doors should also have security stickers.

The Invisible Dog

If you have a dog, great. Dogs can definitely add another layer of protection to your home. Whether or not you actually have a dog, purchase large dog bowls to be displayed near your front and back door. This is one of the easiest and most effective home security tips I can give you. Dogs are loud. Burglars don't want to deal with your dog. If they think it's even possible you have one, they'll likely skip your house and look for an easier target.

Am I on Camera?

Burglars do not want to be caught on film committing a crime. Real working security cameras are terrific, but it's understandable if this expense isn't in your budget. A terrific backup is a knock-off of the real security camera. What makes the fake effective is that it has a battery-operated red blinking light and looks exactly like the real thing. If criminals see a blinking light, they're not going to waste time wondering whether the camera is real. They're going to get out of there before there's evidence of them actually committing a crime.

A client of mine decided to install fake security cameras. Turns out, not long after he installed his fake cameras, his neighbor's house was burglarized. After the burglary, his neighbor came over and asked if he could please pull the footage from his security cameras so that he could see who broke into his home and give the footage to police. My client stood there for a minute, a bit uncomfortable, before fessing up to the neighbor that his cameras were actually fake. It's certainly possible that the criminal skipped out on his house with the cameras and blinking lights, and opted for the less secure home next door.

The Peephole: You Need to Know Who Is on the Other Side

I hope I don't need to tell you why it's a bad idea to answer the door if you don't know who is there. Honestly, I don't answer the door for anyone. It's not worth it. We don't have anything delivered to our home (not even pizza), and I have our mail delivered to a post office box, so there is little reason anyone I'm not expecting should be ringing my doorbell. A regular, traditional peephole is definitely useful because you can see what's happening outside. Obviously, you have to get very close to the door to use it, and you don't want anyone breaking it down. If you're up for making a larger hole in your door, there are great peepholes that allow you to see who is outside from ten feet away. You don't even have to get close to your door. Just remember, if you're not installing a peephole, you've got to know who is on the other side before you open that door by looking through one of your windows.

You Can't Just Ignore It

While I firmly believe you should never open a door unless you know who is there, it's also important that you don't just ignore it. Criminals will often ring your doorbell to determine whether you are home. If you are, they might ask you if you want work done on your house (you don't). A friend of mine heard repeated, insistent knocking on her front door shortly after she moved into her house in New Jersey. She didn't know the guy who was there, and in her gut she felt like something was wrong. She called the police, but in the meantime the knocking got louder. She yelled through the door, "What do you want?" And the guy said, "Oh, is this house for sale?" The second she told him it wasn't, he ran off.

Two men in Colorado Springs are being sought in a rash of daytime burglaries. It is believed that they are breaking into homes after knocking on front doors and ringing doorbells and finding there's no one answering. In Greenwood, Indiana, residents have been urged not to ignore knocks on their doors. A woman at home heard someone knocking on her front door. She ignored it, but then heard a knock at her kitchen door. An individual then tried to break into her front door by ramming it with his shoulder several times. The woman was able to call 911, and the burglar fled the scene.

The Secure Door

So why is it important to have a peephole and a plan of action if there's a knock at the door and you have no idea who it is? The front door is where 70 percent of home invasions occur. For most Americans, a deadbolt on a door that's about three-quarters of an

How to Answer the Door If You Have To

As I've said, I don't answer the door unless I'm expecting friends or family. If there's someone at the door who you aren't expecting, simply speak to the person through the door, and find out what they want. Most front doors aren't soundproof, so you can have a conversation without actually opening the door.

inch thick is all that stands between themselves and a criminal. A horrifying scene unfolded in the home of fifty-nine-year-old Enrique Montes of Phoenix. At about 12:30 a.m., several armed men broke into his home by kicking down the door. The first intruder pointed a gun at Montes. He attempted to push the gun away, and the two began fighting. The fight continued in the home's bedroom, hallway, and kitchen. A second intruder entered the house armed with a rifle and held the other residents in the house hostage. The struggle ended tragically, as Montes was fatally shot in the chest.

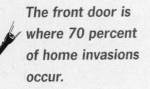

The front door is where 70 percent of home invasions occur.

Terrifying footage of a woman hiding on her roof from an intruder made headlines recently. Melora Rivera climbed out of her second floor window to hide on the roof when she realized there was an intruder in her home. Photos show the young woman crouched under the eaves in her pajamas, while the intruder pops out of a window to look for her. Turns out, a mentally ill homeless man had simply popped out a panel window in her front door, and reached in to unlock it. Luckily the woman was able to grab her phone to call 911 before escaping onto her roof. As both of these stories indicate, having secure doorways is a key component to keeping potential intruders out of your home.

I'm Not the Only One Who Can Pick Your Lock in Under Thirty Seconds

By now, most of my neighbors know about my background. As I've mentioned, this means that when they're locked out, they often ask me to pick their locks for them. I'm pretty good at this, and it's easy for me to do. But guess what? I'm not the only one who can pick a lock. Criminals can do it too. There's an easy way to make this job much more difficult for them—to the point that they'll see your lock and want to skip your house all together. Change your locks. Remember, Kwikset locks, the typical lock you're going to find on a new home, or in apartment buildings, are easy to pick. As you learned in the last chapter, with a bit of practice, you can pick these locks almost as quickly as you could open a door with a key. Invest in a solid sturdy lock, such as the ones made by Schlage or Medeco.

Driveway Alarm

If you live at the end of a long rural driveway, or your house is fairly isolated, a driveway alarm may be a worthwhile security measure for you to take. As crazy as it sounds, it's not unusual for burglars to park right in your driveway. They want quick access to their car for an immediate getaway. Ramona Corrigan of Orange Park, Florida, received an alarming phone call from a neighbor one day. Her neighbor called to let her know that a thief was breaking into her home. Her neighbor had the good sense to call 911 when she saw a truck parked in Corrigan's driveway, and noted the person driving the truck had entered the house. Turns out, the burglar was helping himself to jewelry, cash, a revolver, and Corrigan's father's military medals. Obviously, I'm not suggesting that you need to call the police every time a person uses your driveway to turn around. But if you live in an isolated area, a driveway alarm is a great idea. I also can't stress enough that *if you come home to find a strange car parked in your driveway, do not go into your house.* Call the police, and do not enter your home until you know it is completely safe.

The Safest House on the Block: Safety Measures You Can Take Today

Now that you've cased your house (during the day and at night) and your neighborhood, you can start to implement some of the physical tactics that will help keep your home safe from criminals.

Sight Lines

You want to be sure that you increase visibility throughout your yard as much as possible. There should be no hiding spots. Trees and hedges should be trimmed to a maximum of two to three feet high. Consider pruning trees so that criminals can't climb them to gain access to a second floor or attic.

Lighting

Install motion-activated floodlights around your home. It's a myth that bright lights will help burglars see what they're doing. They don't want you to see them, and bright lights are going to stop them from wanting to rob your house. Make sure that any lights you install are tamper proof.

Secure Your Windows

Most burglars enter a house through the doorway or an open window. Get in the habit of checking regularly that closed windows are locked. Don't assume that just because a family member closed a window that they remembered to lock it. Window coverings are key. At night, no one should be able to see into your home. You don't want a criminal to be able to look directly into your window to see whether you are home. Using landscaping gravel under windows helps eliminate a burglar's ability to creep silently near your home. The crunching sound could alert you to the fact that someone may be outside. Tara Nicole, a woman who took my Spy Escape and Evasion training, suffered greatly as a child because of an open window. Tara was kidnapped through her open bedroom window when she was six years old. All Tara remembers is waking up in the hospital surrounded by

At night, no one should be able to see into your home.

stuffed animals. The kidnapper had slit her throat and left her to die on the side of the road. Tara was lucky; years later it was discovered that her kidnapper had abducted seven other children. The last one he kidnapped he killed.

Use Extra Caution

- Doggy doors are dangerous and not worth the convenience. It's too easy for a criminal to slip into your house through one.

- Secure air-conditioner units. A criminal can pop out a window unit quickly and have immediate access to your home.

- Fences will not protect you. Fences are great for helping keep pets and children safe. However, a fence is easy to open, and takes no time to climb. Unless your fence is thirty feet high, it's not going to keep you or your family safe.

There's an Intruder—Now What?

Trust me, you don't want to wait until you actually suspect someone has broken into your home to think about what to do. You don't want to have to figure out how to protect your family when you hear the sound of glass breaking. It's crucial that you have a solid home defense plan, and it's also important that you take the time to practice it. Let me tell you about my home defense plan, which as you may remember worked great the one time I thought someone might be breaking in. If I hear a suspicious sound, or our alarm system goes off:

What I'll Be Doing
1. I'll grab my flashlight, open my quick-opening safe and grab my gun.

2. I'll run to the top of the stairs, because the stairs are our choke point. This is the place where a criminal will be forced to pass if he is to get to my wife and kids.
3. I'm going to tell the intruder I've called 911 and I have gun.
4. If the criminal is foolish enough to come up the stairs to attack me and my family I will do what's necessary to stop him.

What My Wife Will Be Doing
1. My wife is going to call 911.
2. Then she's going to try and get our children and herself in the same room while I'm at the top of the stairs blocking the choke point.

Keep It Simple

A good home defense plan should be simple and quick. When someone is breaking into your house, your heart is going to be pounding—and research now shows that your brain loses IQ points during stress. Strong emotions such as fear, anxiety, or anger (technically, joy too) sets off the amygdala and impairs the working memory of the prefrontal cortex. This is why it's easy to be overwhelmed in an intensely stressful situation. Thankfully this is only temporary, but again, you don't want to overcomplicate your home defense plan and forget something critical that may cost you your life. Your home defense plan should include three basic tactics:

- Flashlight and weapon (I use a gun, but you could use a knife, bat, or other blunt object).

My Home Defense Nightstand

There's nothing worse than the idea of being violated in your own home. I currently have a few things on my nightstand to help me stop a home invasion should someone try to break in. There's nothing fancy about my nightstand. It's about twenty-four by eighteen inches. Right on top is my Gunvault MV500-STD Microvault. In my gun safe is a loaded Sig Sauer P226. Attached to this gun is a Viridian laser/light combination, model C5L. I also keep a spare magazine in the safe. There is a dedicated prepaid cell phone on my nightstand as well. That phone is always there so that I have at least one cell phone for an emergency call. If I add my regular cell phone to the table I have a backup. You should have one working flashlight available at all times. I happen to have four. (I really like flashlights, if you haven't already noticed.) I have the Surefire 6PX Pro, a Nex-Torch TA1, and an Olight T10, along with my Spy Flashlight. In my experience, all of these flashlights have worked well. This is a simple setup that gives me what I need in case my home alarm goes off in the middle of the night and I have to act fast to protect my family.

- Family member who calls 911.
- A chokepoint (defense position) where you will go to make sure that nobody gets past you.

Where to Safely Store Valuables in Your House

About 95 percent of criminals head straight to the master bedroom. Criminals know that the master bedroom is where cash and jewelry are most likely to be kept. That's why the master bedroom is absolutely the worst place to keep these things. You should be creative about where you keep your cash and valuables in your house. That being said, it's not a bad idea to leave a decoy in the master bedroom. Keeping one piece of jewelry or maybe $20 to $50 in cash might lead the burglar to think he got everything.

Books and Pantries: The DIY Solution

So where should you keep your money? Believe it or not, even though it sounds corny, the hollowed out book is a perfectly good place to keep your cash. I have lots of books in my home, and there's no way a burglar is going to take the time to open and search each book for money. You can buy these books online, or easily make one yourself by taking a razor blade and hollowing out a few pages. Another safe DIY money storage trick is the hollowed out can. Simply take a can opener and open up the bottom of a can of vegetables—something you have a lot of in your pantry or cupboard. Do not remove the bottom of the can, just open it. Use a fork or a butter knife to pry the bottom open, and insert your money. The can will appear untampered with, and a criminal isn't going to go through your entire pantry looking for suspicious cans.

My Partner Travels Frequently for Work. What Can I Do to Make Sure I Keep My Family Safe When I'm Home Alone?

The simplest thing you can do is to get an alarm system. Some people don't realize that you can still use your alarm system while you're at home during the day. Security systems have a "stay" or "home mode" feature. This basically means that the motion detectors are off, so you can move about freely. However, the alarm is going to go off should someone open the door or a window. You'll know immediately if someone has broken into your home while you're inside during the day.

If you're home alone (with or without children), be sure to practice the same security measures that are part of your security routine. Make sure the door is locked, and double-check that all of your windows are closed and locked. Make sure you bring in your mail and newspapers and that your garbage cans aren't left on the street.

Fireproof Protection

If you want to keep valuables safe from fire, fireproof safes are affordable and easy to find. Many of them are small and are perfect for documents, cash, and jewelry. That being said, there's nothing to stop that burglar from simply picking up your safe and walking away with whatever's inside. If you go for this option, choose a model that can be bolted to the floor, or find a creative place to hide your safe. You might want to keep it in a box in the attic marked "old clothes," or "books." Whatever you do, remember, don't keep your fireproof safe in your master bedroom.

If you have a gun safe, this can also be a great place to store valuables. However, do not keep your gun safe somewhere conspicuous, like near the front door. It is also crucial that your gun safe be securely bolted to the floor.

6

TRAVEL SAFETY

Staying Safe in Planes, Taxis, and Hotels

After JetBlue flight 1416 lost its right engine, the cabin began to fill with smoke, and passengers could no longer see the people seated next to them. Passenger Jonathon Hubbard told CNN that he realized he would "have a hard time breathing soon" but oxygen masks did not drop down. Flight attendants went around and deployed them by hand. The plane made a sharp turn back toward the airport. Passengers described how the plane was quaking, and people were crying, terrified by what was happening. Fortunately, the pilot was able to land the plane safely, and only four people were injured. A Southwest Airlines flight from Sacramento, California, made an emergency landing in Los Angeles after the wing flaps malfunctioned. An American Airlines flight headed to Dallas circled in the sky for two hours to burn off fuel so that it could make an emergency landing after the plane blew a tire on takeoff. Even though these types of incidents happen, air travel remains the safest form of travel. If you are flying with a major airline, you have about a 1 in 4.7 million chance of being killed. That being said, incidents happen beyond crashes that you need to be prepared for, such as emergency landings (which can be just as deadly). In the unlikely event there is ever an emergency situation when you are traveling on a plane, there are some tactics you can use to increase your chances of getting out alive.

Ninety Seconds to Safety

We've all seen horrible footage of the aftermath of plane crashes. Based on what most of us have seen on the news, it's easy to assume that all crashes are equally deadly, and you have no chance of surviving whatsoever. The truth is, most passengers don't die from the impact of the crash, but from the smoke inhalation that takes place in fires after impact. In 2005, an Air France Airbus overran the runway in Toronto. The post-crash fire was serious, but all 309 passengers escaped. There were no life-threatening injuries. By the time emergency response teams arrived at the scene, most of the passengers had already managed to exit the aircraft via evacuation slides. The FAA requires that all of a plane's passengers must be able to be evacuated in *ninety seconds*. This small amount of time represents the approximate amount of time you have to get out before you are likely to die from smoke inhalation or fire.

In December 2012, there were only two fatalities in a crash in Rangoon that resulted in the complete burning of a plane. A German journalist who was on board described how he felt the landing gear go down and everything was fine. But suddenly, people were shouting and crying in panic. "A few seconds later, there was fire at the back and out the front. Black smoke filled the plane, and I couldn't breathe or see anything anymore and I realized that something really bad was happening." The journalist recalls the incident happening very quickly, with only about thirty seconds passing between hitting the ground and smoke filling the cabin. The emergency exits were opened by the cabin crew. The passengers all escaped, and the plane burned completely within three minutes. Unfortunately, not all emergencies have such positive endings.

In February 1991, a USAir 737 and a SkyWest commuter plane collided at Los Angeles International Airport. Tragically, everyone on board the commuter plane was killed. While the majority of the passengers on the 737 survived the collision, twenty-two of the passengers died as flames and smoke took over the plane, and it was believed that seventeen of those passengers were making their way to the exits when they were killed by the smoke. James Burnett, the head of the National Transportation Safety Board investigative team, told *People* magazine, "I can't think of a recent accident where this many people have been up out of their seats and didn't make it out." Chaos took over, and people were piled up near a rear exit, desperately trying to get out. The exit was blocked eight or nine people deep. While the tragic outcome of this event was investigated heavily by authorities, and changes are continually being made to improve outcomes in the case of crashes and fires, there are some tactics you can take to increase your chances of survival in a crash, emergency landing, or fire.

Don't Freeze, *Move*

With only ninety seconds to exit a plane in an emergency, it's obviously crucial that you act immediately and quickly. It's hard to believe, but when faced with a life or death situation, it's not uncommon to completely freeze. This is yet another example of how normalcy bias causes us trouble. Dwayne Bennett, who was twenty-seven at the time of the USAir collision, recalled to *People* that as he was trying to escape, he heard a woman shout, "Help me, I can't get out." She was so panicked she was unable to unbuckle her own seat belt. This is not an uncommon reaction.

Floy Olson and her husband, Paul Heck, a retired middle-school teacher, overcame normalcy bias and survived the worst aircraft disaster in history. In 1977, 582 people died when two 747 jumbo jets collided in the Canary Islands. Ten years after the crash, Olson recounted her experience to the *Los Angeles Times*. She credits her husband's quick reaction with saving her life. "I was in shock, and I would have perished if it hadn't been for my husband. I heard a woman shout, 'We've been bombed!' That's what I thought, and I thought I was dying. I heard my husband shout, 'Floy, unfasten your seat belt. Let's get out!'" Olson and Heck made it onto the wing, but were forced to jump two stories to safety. Olson hit her head and lost consciousness for a few minutes. She managed to force herself to crawl away from the plane before it exploded. Olson also told the *Los Angeles Times* that she was never afraid during her escape. She recounted, "I've often wondered why. I didn't have fear, and I can't explain it because I'm a very emotional person. . . . I just knew I had to keep going." No one can predict how they will feel in the face of such an emergency, but with ninety seconds until the fire burns throughout the entire plane, you must motivate yourself and your family to move immediately.

Leave It Behind

It should go without saying, but the brain behaves oddly in emergencies—so tell yourself to leave all personal items behind. In the USAir collision, a woman's purse got caught in the exit. She insisted on taking it because she was afraid of losing her credit cards. Another passenger expressed regret at leaving her violin inside the plane (miraculously, the violin was found later, still intact). In the crash in Rangoon, the German journalist tried to take her carry-on with her. She was concerned about being without a passport. Of course we all know that ultimately physical things such as musical instruments and passports aren't as important as our own lives—but when you're faced with disaster, it's entirely possible you'll have to take a moment to remind yourself to leave all else behind and just move.

The Five-Row Rule

People often believe that the safest place to sit in a plane is in the back—that may be true if the plane hits nose first. Some crashes are tail first, and in that case you obviously wouldn't want to be in the back of the plane. To give yourself the best chances of survival in a crash or in an emergency landing, you want to maximize your chances of getting off the plane in time to escape smoke and fire. Sitting within five rows of an exit maximizes your chances of getting out of the plane alive. Even better than five rows from the exit? Obviously, the exit row itself. Booking an aisle seat is also preferable.

The fewer people you have to deal with to get to an exit the better. The beauty of the Internet age is that when you book your flight online you get to choose your seat. So remember the five-row rule.

Plus Three, Minus Eight

Plus three, minus eight refers to the essential first three minutes after the plane takes off, and last eight minutes of the flight until the plane lands. According to flight crash investigators, most crashes happen during those time periods. In order to increase your chances of survival during takeoff and landing:

- Make it a point to be vigilant. Stay alert. In other words don't immediately fall asleep before takeoff and make sure you're awake before landing.
- Keep your shoes on. It's also a good idea to think about traveling in comfortable, secure shoes (not sandals).
- Don't let yourself be encumbered or distracted by devices or reading materials.
- If you drink, skip preflight cocktails; it's not worth it.
- Make sure your seat belt is securely fastened.
- Note exits and your exact distance from them by counting seats.

Read the Safety Card

If you're like most people, you're busy looking at your tablet or smartphone or reading the paper while the flight attendants are doing their safety checks. It's easy to assume you know everything you need to know—you've heard the speech about how to fasten seat belts and what to do if the oxygen tanks come down many times before. However, it's important to familiarize yourself with the safety card each time you fly. Planes are different, and as you now know, it's essential to know where the exits are in an emergency situation. You also want to remind yourself what the brace position is, and to know how exactly your seat cushion would work if you needed to use it as a flotation device. I realize that only about 1 percent of you will actually read the safety card, but it takes only about two minutes to read over.

Pre-Takeoff Checklist
- Count number of seats from your row to the nearest exit.
- Take note of the surroundings. Are there any potential obstacles you'd have to deal with in an emergency?
- Keep your shoes on.
- Keep your seat belt tightly fastened.
- Read the emergency card.
- Check for your flotation device.
- Stay awake.

Taxis Are Not as Safe as You Think

Most people who travel for pleasure or business get off the plane and into a taxi. It's actually the taxi ride that is the more dangerous part of your journey. Many of us also feel safer taking a taxi back home or to our hotel after a night out on the town or we take taxis to avoid walking alone late at night. Whatever the reason you take a taxi, there are some crucial steps you must take to stay safe.

In New York City, a taxi driver was recently sentenced to

twenty years for raping a female passenger. A twenty-nine-year-old dozed off in the backseat of the taxi and woke up to find herself being assaulted by her driver. She was restrained, and held at knife-point. In Kansas City, a woman says she was sexually assaulted and robbed by a taxi driver. She was intoxicated and opted to take a taxi home after going out to bars. A man posing as a cab driver tried to rape a woman in front of her three young children in Queens, New York. Authorities stated that there was nothing to indicate that the man was a licensed livery cab driver.

Taxis are dangerous.

Taxis are dangerous. When you get in a taxi you are putting yourself in a vulnerable position. You have no idea who you've just gotten into a car with, and you are trusting a total stranger with your safety and well-being. Foreign taxis can be especially dangerous. A young Australian woman survived a month of hiking in the Andes mountains in South America only to be shot by a taxi driver in a botched robbery. Elizabeth Littlewood and her boyfriend were on their way to the airport when they jumped into what they thought was a normal taxi. When the driver asked them for money in Spanish, the pair did not understand what he was saying. Elizabeth thought the driver wanted her to exit the taxi. She was shot in the stomach when she tried to open the door handle.

Don't Fall for Taxi Scams

I've outlined worst-case scenario situations for taxis, because I believe in being informed and safe. I also want you to enjoy family vacations and have successful business trips, so I also think you should be familiar with common scams that take place in taxis. In

Las Vegas, "long hauling," or taking tourists on the longest route possible, has become a serious problem. A Las Vegas taxi driver who has been driving for fourteen years spoke to the *Las Vegas Review Journal*, describing the problem as "truly epidemic" and explaining that taxi drivers were "coming up with more creative ways to take people on longer rides." A state audit showed that nearly one in four passengers were taken on purposely longer rides than necessary. Luckily this is not a life-or-death situation, but you are still getting ripped off.

A Washington, DC–area man recently pleaded guilty to a scheme in which he posed as a taxi driver, picked up young, intoxicated people and scammed them out of their money. Nyerere Mitchell convinced passengers to let him use their ATM cards to take out money for their fares. He would purposely use ATMs where the machine could be used only on the driver's side. He'd use the passenger's card, taking out much more money than the ride cost. Mitchell managed to steal more $200,000 from more than sixty DC residents.

In New York City, thousands of taxi drivers overcharged passengers by putting the meter on "suburban rate" rather than the standard rate. This cost passengers an estimated $8.3 million in just two years. In one particularly extreme example, a cabbie picked up an eighteen-year-old college student at O'Hare airport in Chicago. The student was from China, and spoke little English. The cab driver told the student there were no buses available to take the student from O'Hare airport to Champaign, but that he would take him there for "the low price of $1,000." Once the taxi arrived at Champaign, the driver demanded $4,800 from the student. While the student didn't have that much cash, he handed over every penny he had to the taxi driver.

When a Taxi Is Your Only Option

While there are many hardworking taxi drivers out there who aren't out to rip you off or harm you in any way, it's in your best interest to be informed and aware of situations in which someone can take advantage of you. Once again, I'll remind you that situational awareness is key. You want to be aware of your surroundings, and you never want to get into a car with a stranger if you're impaired in any way. If you have no other choice than to take a taxi to get to your destination, there are a few basic rules you should always follow.

Know Where You're Going

Familiarize yourself with the best route to your destination. Rather than depend on a stranger to get you from point A to point B, tell him exactly what route you'd like to take. Pay attention to where he's driving, and know if he is veering off your preplanned route. Tell him immediately to return to the correct route. Get out of the car if he doesn't comply with your instructions.

Do Your Research

While it's essential to stay alert regardless of where you travel, it can be helpful to know what kinds of scams take place in the particular country you are traveling to. For instance, in Buenos Aires, drivers have been known to give a "fake bill." A driver will accept a tourist's bill, then swap them for a counterfeit and tell the passenger they can't accept their money. Travel bloggers warn tourists traveling to this area to pay in exact change and be alert when using Mex$100 and Mex$50 notes. In the Dominican Republic, there are reports of Americans getting into taxis without air-conditioning at the airport. The driver will roll down the window, and when the car stops at a traffic light, a motorcyclist will reach in and steal whatever they can get their hands on. It's also helpful to know what is standard behavior when taking taxis when you travel. It's perfectly acceptable to hail a taxi from the street in New York City, but that might not be the case in Taiwan. Research reputable taxi companies, and keep their phone number with you at all times. Also, when overseas, always ask the hotel you are staying at to call a taxi for you, and ask which cab companies you can trust.

Only You Decide Where You're Going

Do not allow a taxi driver (or anyone) to talk you out of going to your original destination. You never want to be in a situation where the driver has complete control—and you don't know where you're going. Do not allow a driver to suggest alternative hotels, restaurants, clubs, or bars, and never trust him if he's "taking you on a shortcut" to save you money. It's likely possible he's working in conjunction with another person from the establishment—and recommending it for a fee. Deviating from your original plan also puts you in the dangerous position of not knowing where you are or if your taxi driver is going the right way.

Is It Legit?

Before getting into a taxi it's essential you check for a few simple things: (1) The doors should have handles on the inside. If there is no way for you to get out of the taxi on your own, do not get in. (2) Be sure there is a picture of the driver, the medallion is posted, and the taxi has a radio. If any of these items is missing, do not get in the taxi. (3) Make sure you've picked up the taxi at a legitimate taxi stand. Don't take a ride from the guy who is standing against the wall in the airport saying, "You need a ride?"

Taxis Are Not for Sharing

It might seem like a good idea to share a taxi with someone. You might think it will cut down on your waiting time at a busy airport or that it makes sense if you're in a place where finding a taxi is difficult. Obviously, it's also cheaper. Sharing a taxi with a stranger puts you in a vulnerable position. The person you are riding with might have an alternative agenda or could be working in conjunction with the driver.

It's become increasingly popular to use apps that provide customers with rides in private cars. According to the *Daily Beast*, there have been questions about whether such services keep the customer's information private. Women have reported receiving text messages and messages via Facebook from drivers. Some women report that the only way drivers could have gotten in touch with them is if their driver was given their personal information when they booked the ride. Think twice about getting in a car that's operated by a technology company and might not use the same background checks and undertake the same security measures as other taxi companies do.

Don't Jump at Your First Option

After a long trip, it's natural to want to get away from the airport or train station and to your destination as quickly as possible. However, jumping in the first taxi you see is a big mistake and can really get your trip off on the wrong foot. Airports and busy train stations often attract unofficial taxis, and it's best to stick with an area-licensed official taxi. Never opt for jumping in a taxi because the driver is available and you want to avoid a long line at a taxi stand. If it's not immediately clear how to access a taxi from the airport, find the transportation desk and get instructions. It's also a good idea to inquire about general prices or find out approximate costs in advance of your trip.

Windows Up

It can be really tempting to open the windows and enjoy the breeze, especially when you've just started your vacation. When riding in taxis, the rule of thumb is, windows up—or just slightly cracked if absolutely necessary. Criminals are on the lookout for easy targets, and you don't want to advertise that you're an easy target by opening your window. Thieves can easily reach in and grab your belongings as the car slows or stops at a red light. Of course, you should never roll down your window if someone on the street gestures for you to do so.

Be Discreet

Again, this goes back to situational awareness. Don't spend your taxi ride sending texts on your smartphone. Smartphones are easy to steal and attract thieves. You'll also want to think twice about wearing expensive jewelry or watches. I'm not saying you need to dress like a slob when you travel, just that you should be aware of displaying valuables that will tempt criminals.

Drew avoided a potentially dangerous situation after taking my class. Drew was on the holiday of a lifetime with his wife and adult son and daughter. They were traveling to Scotland, England, Holland, and France. When they arrived at the Paris train station, Drew's knowledge of travel safety and situational awareness came in very handy. He describes exiting the train station and encountering crazy crowds. It was not immediately clear where the taxi stands were located. Drew's wife and daughter got separated from him in the crowd, and before he could catch up to them a man appeared asking his wife if she needed a cab. She said yes and further explained that they would need a large taxi, because they had lots of bags and were a large group. The man replied with a big smile that he had just the thing. Drew's wife felt that she had had a stroke of good luck. The man grabbed her bag and started moving quickly out of the station. He urged his son and daughter to follow. Drew said his alertness level immediately went up. He felt this situation was too easy, too quick, and too lucky. He felt if it was too good to be true, it's probably trouble. Drew decided to focus and get serious about what was happening. He chased them around a corner where he found his family being led to a large unmarked van. An imposing, unfriendly man was waiting at the van, and he told the family they should get in the van, and that he would load their bags for them. Drew checked for his tactical pen, and said firmly, "No. This doesn't feel right, get our bags back now." Drew's son began to wrestle the bag back from the larger man. Drew started asking questions: "Where is your license? Where is your taxi light on the vehicle? Where is your meter?" The smaller man kept smiling, and tried to convince them they were a "special private taxi" and that the family should feel lucky they spotted them. Drew's wife unfortunately did not share his sense of concern and didn't want to drag the bags back to the long taxi line. Drew felt very strongly that this was not an official cab, and they were potentially entering into a very dangerous situation. Drew feels that his family really dodged a bullet, and at the very least they would have ended up a long way from their hotel with a huge bill. The real taxi line was thirty minutes long, and Drew had to pay for two taxis to fit his family and all of their belongings, but they ended up at their destination safely. Drew's instincts were abso-

You're Trapped in the Back of a Taxi and Need to Get Out. What Would You Do?

First, I'd try to open the door to see if I could roll out at a stop-light. If the doors were locked, I'd have to kick open a window. To easily kick out a window you want to lie on your back. You're going to use the force of both legs to break the glass at the lower right portion of the window—where it's going to be easi-est to break it. Keep your legs together, and start kicking that part of the window with both of your feet until the glass breaks. In this kind of situation, you've got to remember that the glass is tighter in the corners, so that's where you'll have a better chance of breaking it. If you kick the center of the window, your feet are going to bounce right off. To watch a video of me dem-onstrating this, visit SpySecretsBook.com.

lutely correct. This situation was full of red flags, and thanks to his knowledge of travel safety and good use of situational aware-ness, his family was able to continue enjoying their vacation safely.

Hotel Safety

We'd all like to believe we're safe when sleeping soundly in a hotel room, but that's not necessarily the case. The boxer Mike Tyson woke up to rustling in his hotel room at the Cosmopolitan of Las

Vegas. Luckily for the intruder, he escaped before Tyson realized what was actually happening. In Orlando, Florida, a woman was crying and screaming and pounding on the door of a hotel room at a Super 8. The men inside looked through the peephole, and saw the upset woman who they believed needed help. They opened the door, and several men entered the room and robbed the victims at gunpoint. During a string of robberies in an Orlando-area hotel district, a tourist was shot when returning from Walt Disney World. The tourist and his brother were pushed into their second story hotel room by the robbers. In Hyannis, Massachusetts, an elderly couple from Pennsylvania were robbed at knifepoint shortly after checking in to their hotel rooms. They were unlocking their room door when a man pushed it open and forced his way in. Mike McGowan, seventy-eight, ended up in a wrestling match with the robber. McGowan was flipped onto his stomach while the knife was held to him and his wallet was stolen.

Hotels and Fires

Fires in hotels are also a cause for concern. Ten years after surviving the MGM Grand Hotel fire, the second worst hotel fire in American history, survivor Rafael Patino shared his story with the *Los Angeles Times*. On November 21, 1980, eighty-four people died and 679 were injured after the fire started with an electrical issue in a ground-floor restaurant. The blaze quickly spread due to the presence of combustible materials and a lack of fire sprinklers. Roy L. Parrish, the fire chief at the time, said that four minutes after the fire left the restaurant, it hit the lobby's front doors and blew out all the glass. The fire was traveling at seventeen feet per second.

Patino and his wife, who were at the hotel for a convention, were staying on the sixteenth floor. They realized their hotel was on fire only after looking out the window. There were no alarms or sprinklers to indicate that something was wrong. The Patinos left their room but were confronted by a wall of black smoke so thick that they briefly lost each other. Luckily, unlike many other guests who left their rooms, Mr. Patino had kept his room key and was able to get back in. The couple recalled their harrowing experience of stuffing towels under the door to stave off smoke, and hiding under a tent made out of curtains on their balcony. Glass was being blown out of windows, and they huddled on the balcony for more than two hours while waiting to be rescued. The Patinos were eventually rescued, but many others were not as lucky. The majority of the victims died between the nineteenth and twenty-fourth floors, where most of the smoke had risen through elevator shafts and air-conditioning ducts.

Obviously, hotels are often a necessary part of travel—whether it's for business or pleasure. I'm not suggesting that your family not take vacations due to the potential dangers of hotels or that you stop traveling for your job.

I've been lucky enough to travel to places like France, Italy, Switzerland, Austria, and Greece. And I meet lots of wonderful people traveling across the country teaching my Spy Escape and Evasion classes. However, I always make a point to follow some very basic but important safety rules when staying in a hotel. I am also sure to have a few items with me to help ensure my safety.

How to Enjoy a Safe Hotel Stay

Where to Book Your Room

‣ Stay between floors three and six. Criminals target the first two floors because they can quickly rob the rooms and then have quick access to a getaway car. You don't want to stay higher than the sixth floor because in the United States a fire truck ladder will reach only to the sixth floor. If there's a fire and you're on the seventy-seventh floor, you've got a long way to get down.

‣ Do not stay near a stairwell. Criminals will often target rooms next to the stairwells since they provide easy access to escape.

‣ Practice situational awareness and make sure you are not followed off of the elevator. Should you ever suspect you are being followed off the elevator, do not enter your room. Call for help. Depending on the severity of the situation and what your gut tells you, you might call the front desk or the police.

Protect Yourself and Your Belongings

‣ Do not forget to use your lock. The second you walk into your room, lock the door.

‣ Use a door alarm stopper. This is a very inexpensive security item that can save your vacation—if not your life. Simply set the alarm in front of your door while you're in your room, and it will be set off automatically if someone opens your door, resulting in an extremely loud noise.

Hotel Room Fire Protection

‣ Locate the exits. Before settling into your room, find the exits and note how many doors down the exits are. Note if you have to turn a corner, and which way you would have to go. You want to be able to locate the exits quickly even if you are unable to see.

‣ Consider investing in smoke hoods and gas masks. This is crucial if you need to travel to a third-world country. This is what executive protection agents carry with them when protecting people in certain overseas areas.

‣ Bring a hotel escape bag. This is a simple, light bag containing a few essential items that can save your life. A hotel escape bag usually contains about fifty feet of rope (about ten feet per floor), gloves for rope burn, and a carabiner that can support a weight of around thirteen hundred pounds. This is all you really need to get yourself safely out of a hotel room. In the event you needed to escape, you would clip your carabiner around a heavy piece of furniture (or around door hinges), and then use the rope to ease yourself to safety through a window.

Think Twice About Your Vacation Destination

The last thing you want to do on vacation is worry about violent crime. Vacations are meant to be a time of fun and relaxation, so I highly recommend that you think carefully about booking vacations in certain areas. While it's always important to familiarize yourself with areas you are traveling to, some places have simply become too dangerous for American travelers, in my opinion. These destinations include Mexico, which is currently the kidnapping capital of the world and also known for carjacking, high-way robbery, and robbery by organized criminal groups, and the Caribbean—particularly Jamaica, which has one of the highest per capita murder rates in the world.

While there are undeniably many wonderful places to visit in the Caribbean and Mexico, it's really important that you understand the dangers of traveling to such places. Just because you are staying in a beautiful, well-run resort, doesn't mean that the crime and poverty these countries are suffering from ceases to exist. Educate yourself about potential hazards when making travel plans, and as always, practice situational awareness at all times.

7

HOW TO RUN
COUNTERSURVEILLANCE
LIKE A PRO

Many people are familiar with the Cheshire murders, the tragic home invasion that took the lives of Jennifer Hawke Petit, forty-eight, and her two daughters, ages eleven and seventeen. Mrs. Petit had been shopping with Michaela at the local ShopRite when career criminal Joshua Komisarjevsky noticed a large diamond ring on her finger. Komisarjevsky followed Mrs. Petit and her daughter as they shopped, and then followed them out to their car. Komisarjevsky proceeded to follow the Petits to their comfortable suburban home. Later that night, Komisarjevsky met up with another career criminal. The pair walked into an open door of the Petit house, where they assaulted and murdered the two girls and their mother. Mr. Petit was the only survivor.

The Petit family was well respected and revered in their community. They had no reason to believe that anyone would wish to do them harm. Unfortunately, the Petit tragedy illustrates how dangerous a situation can be when a criminal believes (whether it's true or not) that you have something they desperately want.

Criminals will often follow, observe, or stalk their victims in advance of committing a crime. In most kidnappings, muggings, and home invasions, the victim has been under surveillance from anywhere from a few minutes to a couple of hours to a few days or weeks. In New York City, a sexual predator attacked a woman after following her home from the Grand Concourse in the Bronx. In North Carolina, a woman was followed home by a man who was behind her in traffic, claiming he needed to warn her of damage to her vehicle. He pushed his way into her apartment and sexually assaulted her before she could lock the door. All of these incidents are tragic, and have undoubtedly caused intense trauma and heartache for the victims and their families. Fortunately, I've successfully taught thousands of people to run countersurveillance and to determine quickly and easily if they are being followed. Having the skills and capabilities to know you are under surveillance is empowering. Being aware that you are being followed provides the essential opportunity to take action to secure your safety.

What Exactly Is Surveillance?

When you think of surveillance the average person probably imagines a couple of guys parked in a van with video equipment, doughnuts, and lots of coffee. Or maybe the word *surveillance* makes you think of the many security cameras you encounter throughout the day. What exactly is surveillance? Surveillance is used to monitor behavior, activities, or any other information that may change.

Surveillance is generally used to influence, manage, or protect people. There are many different types of surveillance that the average person comes in contact with. Most of us are used to seeing cameras that record activity everywhere from stadiums and airports to restaurants and schools. We've all heard of the surveillance that takes place on social networks such as Facebook and Twitter, where information is used to create maps of social networks and the data are mined for useful information about possible terrorists. Just some of the many other forms of surveillance include corporate surveillance, profiling, aerial, and biometric surveillance. For example, I'm the CEO of a company called Global Protection and Intelligence. We're an executive protection and investigations firm. We're often hired by celebrities to run surveillance on spouses or lovers who might be cheating on them.

Without years of painstaking surveillance work, Osama Bin Laden would never have been killed. The hunt for Osama Bin Laden (also known by his code name "Geronimo") involved interrogation of CIA detainees in secret prisons, eavesdropping on telephone calls and emails, the collection of 387 high-resolution and infrared images of the Abbottabad compound, installing spyware and tracking devices, a fleet of satellites collecting electronic signals over Pakistan, advanced drones, and even a team of CIA agents sequestered in a rented house to determine if Bin Laden was really there. And on May 2, 2011, after using every surveillance tactic the U.S. government had, CIA director Leon Panetta was able to announce to the president and his advisers gathered in the situation room at the White House: "Geronimo EKIA." Or, Osama Bin Laden—Enemy Killed in Action.

The capture of Osama Bin Laden is obviously an extreme example of what can be accomplished with high-quality surveillance tactics. What we are concerned with is the surveillance a criminal may use on you.

Most Crimes Are Crimes of Opportunity

The average American may think that they don't have a real reason to run surveillance or countersurveillance, except maybe to see if their teenage son is really going where he says he's going. However, as the previous stories indicate, it's very common for a criminal to follow a victim home and wait for the perfect moment to break into your home and rob you—or worse.

Brad Heath's article "The Ones That Get Away" for *USA Today* shed light on a terrifying development in law enforcement. Police and prosecutors are allowing tens of thousands of wanted felons to go free by simply crossing a state border. *USA Today* uncovered that approximately 3,300 of these individuals were accused of sexual assaults, robberies, and homicides. Police in high-crime cities, including Atlanta, Little Rock, and Philadelphia, have told the FBI that they would not pursue 90 percent of their suspects into other states. *USA Today* discovered that among the individuals who would not be pursued are a Florida man who hacked his roommate's neck with a machete after a fight over a can of beer and two of Pittsburgh's most wanted fugitives. I'm not suggesting that you live your life in fear of these criminals who have found a way to escape justice at the expense of society. However, I do believe that by arming yourselves with my Spy Escape and Evasion tactics, you'll be able to keep yourself and your family safe from violent criminals.

Remember, most crimes are crimes of opportunity. This means that criminals are looking for the perfect circumstances under which to commit their crime. By arming yourself with the simple basics of surveillance you can do your best to ensure that you will not fit the picture of a criminal's ideal victim.

Would You Know If You Were Being Followed?

Do you think you would know if you were being followed? Chances are, unless you're using my Spy Escape and Evasion techniques, you wouldn't. Every year my college buddies and I meet in Las Vegas for the March Madness basketball tournament. We have a great time—a big group of guys hanging out, watching multiple games on multiple screens, and eating an insane amount of hot dogs. One year, my friend Adam kept getting up and leaving while we were watching one of the games. He was also acting strangely, not giving a direct answer about where he was going, and he would almost stutter before giving us the answer, "I'm going to the bathroom." Finally, I decided to follow him to see what was up. I followed him all the way through the casino, and he never saw me. I kept my distance, using the slot machines as cover and having plenty of patience in my pursuit. Eventually I followed him to the Sports Book. It turned out he had placed a bet on another game and he kept going out to check on his bet. He didn't tell us where he was really going because his bet was doing badly, and he definitely knew we'd make fun of him for placing such a terrible bet. Adam had no idea I was following him until I walked up to him in the Sports Book. Thankfully for Adam, I was just a concerned friend and he wasn't in danger of anything except maybe being laughed at. If Adam had any situational awareness, even if he had looked over his shoulder once, he would have seen me. I wasn't exactly trying to be James Bond—I wasn't worried about getting caught, I just wanted to know what he was really up to.

Why Would Anyone Follow Me?

You certainly don't have to be working for the CIA for someone to want to follow you. While it may seem incredibly unlikely that anyone would want to follow you, there are many reasons a person might put you under surveillance. If you were ever involved in a divorce, custody battle, lawsuit or dispute with a coworker, it's possible someone could have gotten angry enough to want to do you harm. It could be something as simple as accidentally taking a parking space that someone else was waiting for, or maybe a criminal has decided that you look like you have money and are worth robbing.

Whatever the reason a person may think he or she has to put you under surveillance, it's best to practice constant awareness, and remain in Condition Yellow to guarantee your safety. In the event you are being followed, chances are that the individual or individuals following you are regular people—a person with a grudge or a common criminal who is looking for some cash for his next drug fix. While that sounds alarming, the good news is that by following a few simple steps, you can easily determine if you are being followed by an amateur. If you figure out that you are under surveillance, you'll be able to take the appropriate measures to avoid a dangerous confrontation.

Am I Actually Being Followed?

A CIA officer knows how crucial it is to run surveillance detection routes if you think you are being followed. While this may sound complicated, it's not actually difficult to do. The following story is a great example of how an average person can run a surveillance detection route to determine whether she is in danger. Hannah, a twenty-something from Brooklyn, clearly remembers the day she was followed. Hannah was looking at handbags in a major department store in a crowded Brooklyn neighborhood. She soon suspected something wasn't quite right. "I noticed a guy hanging around who didn't really seem interested in bags. I thought it was weird, but I brushed it off," she recalls. Still feeling concerned that this person was paying too much attention to her, Hannah decided to walk into the perfume section. "The guy seemed to be following me, but I still thought I was just being paranoid." Hannah wanted to be completely sure that she was being followed, so she decided to go upstairs to the women's shoe section, thinking that if he showed up there, he was definitely following her. Sure enough, the man ended up in the women's shoe department, watching Hannah while he talked on his cell phone. "I felt my heart sink, I started to feel panicky and scared. I started to wonder how long this guy was following me for, had it been all day? What if he had been following me for weeks? I had no idea what to do." Hannah remembers being afraid to make a scene in public, but realized she needed to make a decision not to live in fear and let someone intimidate her. She walked over to the man and said, "Excuse me." Hannah recalls he just turned his head slowly and walked away, refusing to look her in the eye. "After a couple of minutes he was back, so I decided to find a security guard." When the man saw her talking to the security guard, he put his head down and quickly walked out of the store. Luckily Hannah did not encounter the man again, and she's learned to be vigilant about what's happening in her immediate surroundings. Hannah actually ran a perfect surveillance detection route. She went from handbags to perfume to shoes, knowing that if someone traces the same exact path, it's unlikely to be a coincidence. It was clear she was being followed.

Situational Awareness Is the First Step

Like Hannah, if you're focused on your immediate surroundings, it's very likely that you will notice if you are being followed. Keep your head up, stay aware, and make a point to notice the people around you (or cars if you are in your vehicle) at all times. Had Hannah been focusing her attention on texting, or talking on her phone, or engrossed in conversation with a friend, she might have not noticed a man hanging around in the handbag department. He could have followed her throughout the store without her ever knowing. I can't stress enough that if you are not operating in Condition Yellow, you will not notice if a criminal is sizing you up to see if you'll make a good victim. Hannah first became suspicious that she was under surveillance when a man appeared in a section of a store where he didn't seem to belong. She knew the baseline of the handbag section, and it didn't include a lot of male shoppers. This was a good indicator that someone was trying to follow her.

Hannah's experience fits in with a rule of thumb we follow in the intelligence world:

One time = an accident
Two times = a coincidence
Three times = enemy action

Of course, it's entirely possible he could have been looking for a gift for his mom or girlfriend. Hannah wisely ran a "surveillance detection route" by going into women's shoes to confirm the man was following her. Then the man appeared a third time. It became clear he was focusing on Hannah and that she had to take immediate action to remain safe. Speaking to the security guard and staying in a crowded public place was absolutely the right thing to do, denying him the opportunity to continue to follow her further.

> *A person who intends to do you harm will start matching your pacing.*

To ensure that you are not under surveillance, be vigilant. Pay extra attention. A CIA officer would always note the following scenarios:

- **A person walking too close to you on the street:** As I've mentioned, a person who intends to do you harm will start matching your pacing. If you take small steps, he will match your small steps stride per stride. This is a big indicator that something is going to happen.
- **Someone making intense eye contact with you:** If a person is staring you down, this is a sign that something is going to happen. People usually look away when someone meets their stare. That is the normal human reaction.
- **A person who seems way too interested in you:** If someone is appearing at the same place and the same time during your daily routine (school drop off, the coffee shop, the bus stop, the gym), monitor that person and keep an eye on him.

Don't discount any uncomfortable feelings you may have including uneasiness, anxiety, doubt, suspicion, hesitation, or fear.

If one or more of these actions is taking place, it's possible you are under surveillance.

Surveillance in the Car

It's also possible that you'll be followed in your car. You may notice a particular car you've never seen before driving through your neighborhood. Maybe you see a vehicle that's taking the same turns as you on your commute, driving to the grocery store or home. Or you may notice someone driving past you occasionally, then changing lanes and falling back again. To confirm that you are being followed by another car, try the following.

If you're on the highway, get off and then back on. Is the car still behind you when you get back on? Purposefully and carefully slow down. Is the car you think is following you driving at the same pace as you are? For example, if you are driving 75 miles per hour on the highway, slow down to 60. All of the other cars should still pass you, but if the car you believe may be following you also slows down, you know you're being followed.

If you are noticing any of these patterns it's possible you are under surveillance.

I'm Under Surveillance: Now What?

It's not just enough to determine if you're being followed. The person who is pursuing you must be confronted. Helen's story is a perfect example of how powerful this technique can really be.

Helen was running up the hill toward her favorite jogging path when she noticed a man walking with a large dog. She got the feeling that something wasn't right. Soon he was just a short distance behind Helen, who was growing increasingly uncomfortable. "All my red flags and alarm bells went off to say, 'You're not safe, this isn't right,' so I made a decision based on that feeling." Helen stopped, turned around, and deliberately looked directly at the man following her. This signaled to the man that she knew exactly what he was up to. At that point the man quickly turned left and ran into the park, while Helen decided to run directly home along a heavily trafficked road.

Helen did the right thing. She stopped and let the follower know she was aware of what was happening. Had Helen ignored the warning signals and continued into the park, the man could have done her harm once they were in a more secluded area. Helen's acknowledging what was happening caused the man to stop following her and move on. Of course, had the man continued to follow her or make her uncomfortable in any way, she should have immediately called 911. But the fact is, since most crimes are crimes of opportunity, the criminal will most likely go looking for someone else if they know you've spotted them.

There are five simple tactics intelligence officers use to run countersurveillance. You don't need to be a government operative with years of experience to use these steps. They are easy to execute, and may keep you out of serious danger.

Tactic One: The Pause and Turn

When a person is following you with the intent to do you harm, the *pause and turn* can be a very helpful way both to determine if you are under surveillance and to let the person know you are aware of what she's doing. While you are walking, simply pause, turn around, and pretend to do something—like check your phone, tie a shoe, or turn around as if you were looking for someone. Then look directly at the person you think is following you. Your typical amateur who is following you is going to get flustered and give herself away. She's likely to freeze or act unnatural because you have caught her by surprise. In other words, someone who is following you will not exhibit the same natural behavior as someone who is simply walking down the street.

Tactic Two: The Acknowledgment

As I just mentioned, once you have determined that you are being followed, it's important to let the person know that you are aware of what they're doing. Once a potential threat is acknowledged, most criminals will leave you alone. Remember, criminals are looking for ideal victims, and by acknowledging that you are aware of their presence and that they are planning to do you harm makes you a less appealing victim. By seeking the help of the security guard at the department store, Hannah was telling her follower that she was onto him, and not going to tolerate being followed. It was at that point that the man exited the store. A woman I know who was concerned she was being followed into the subway abruptly turned around and said, "What?" to her follower. He turned around and left immediately. Turning around and confidently asking, "Can I help you?" is likely to result in someone choosing to leave you alone.

Tactic Three: Don't Be a Soft Target

Don't be an ideal victim. Exhibit a sense of strength, walk tall, and keep your head up. Call someone and discuss in an obvious and audible manner that there is a person following you. Don't be afraid to have your tactical pen out and ready to use. Remember that when criminals are shown pictures of people they'd attack, they choose people who look weak or like they're not paying attention—with their heads down and shoulders slumped.

Tactic Four: Stay Public

You never want a criminal to know where you live.

If you've determined that someone is following you, it is essential that you do not go home. It may seem like home is a safe place . . . you can lock the doors, call for help—but this is the absolute last place you should go. You never want a criminal to know where you live. The criminal may try to break into your home, or he'll give you the impression that he has gone, when ultimately he is hiding and preparing to break in at a later time. To ensure your safety if you are under surveillance:

- Stay in a crowded, public place, and call for help. Safe places include restaurants, cafes, busy stores, and crowded street corners.
- You never want to walk down an alley or isolated street where you may end up closed off from other people, making it easy for a criminal to hurt you.
- If you're being followed in a public place such as the grocery store, do not attempt to leave the store and get in

Check Their Shoes

If you're on foot and you suspect you are under surveillance, pay attention to the person's shoes to determine if it's the same person who is following you. It's easy to remove or put on a baseball cap, sunglasses, or other items that may quickly make it harder to identify a particular individual. However, it's not as easy to carry around an extra pair of shoes. The shoes a person is wearing will likely remain the same.

your car. All the criminal needs to do is wait at the entrance for you to come out of the store. He can then follow you to your car where he may either confront you or follow you home.

Tactic Five: Slow Down and Mix Things Up

If you've determined that another car is following you, keep driving (again, never go home if a car is following you), change speeds and make multiple turns to let the follower know you are aware of him. When you are able to safely do so, note the make and the license plate number of the car so that you can give this information to the police.

When You Have a High Threat Level

If you have a tumultuous relationship with an ex-husband or a boyfriend who is harassing you all the time—or you've had a disagreement with a former employee or coworker, you may want to proceed as if you have a high threat level. You should also operate on a high threat level if you have suspicions about a person you've been noticing on a regular basis. Is there someone outside the gym every time you leave after a workout? Are you suspicious about someone who seems to get coffee at the same place and the same time as you do? If you are operating on a high-threat level there are a few additional precautions that it's important for you to take.

Change Your Behavior

If you are concerned that a specific person may want to follow you, make a point to continually change your patterns. This can be difficult, as we are creatures of habit and it's hard to break our routines. To ensure your safety, it's crucial that you mix up the routes you take as well as the order of your activities:

- Vary the time you leave the house in the morning.
- Change the route and timing of your commute.
- Mix up your activities. If you buy coffee at the same coffee shop every day, vary your routine so that you're hitting different places at different times.
- Visit restaurants you haven't been to before.
- Take a different route home from work.

It should be noted that while operating with a high threat level does make it more difficult for you to be followed, it's no substitute for practicing constant vigilance. Never stop operating in Condition Yellow. Remember, Condition Yellow keeps you from finding yourself in Condition Red—the crisis condition.

Your Inner Spy

I never imagined my CIA surveillance skills would come in handy after meeting the father of a woman I was dating. Back when I was single, I met a nice girl—and we ended up having a great first date. The second one was good too, and I eventually was invited to meet her father at a dinner party. Before the party, she told me that her father was in the construction business and he used to employ John Gotti, the infamous New York mafia crime boss. The woman I was dating also happened to tell me a story about her parents meeting a notorious hit man. I was starting to get suspicious. While I didn't have any proof that her father was in the mafia—if it walks like a duck and sounds like a duck. . . . I always size people up quickly when I meet them, and I noticed right away that like me, her father had a knife clipped to his pants pocket. When I asked him what kind of knife it was, he jumped back—very alarmed. He asked me immediately if I was carrying a gun. While I usually carry a gun, Maryland's laws didn't allow me to carry my concealed weapon, and I told him so. After this exchange he was perfectly nice, but still struck me as stereotypical mafia—like someone right out of *The Sopranos*. Later that night my girlfriend called me sobbing. Her dad wanted to know why she'd bring an FBI agent to a dinner party. Her dad demanded my name, address, phone number, tags—he wanted to know everything about me. She had already told him I wasn't in the FBI, but he didn't care, and she wanted to give me a heads up. I immediately went on high alert. I started carrying my gun 24/7. I ran surveillance detection routes going to and coming home from work, and I added tons of security measures around the house (alarm system, video cameras, motion detectors). I knew they would probably hire a skip tracer to check me out and make sure I wasn't in the FBI. I knew this process would take a week or two, and I'd have to use all of my surveillance secrets to stay alive.

I was eventually invited back to dinner, so I figured they realized I didn't pose a threat. However, her father asked me to sit down and talk. "Jason, we're going hunting this weekend and we'd like you to join us." No way was I going hunting with the mafia and their ten guns to my one. Obviously the mafia didn't get me; I'm still here. My point is that just when you think all is well, you find out your girlfriend's father is in the mafia, and you're suddenly really glad you have those countersurveillance skills. While I was able to easily handle this situation on my own, more serious situations could have called for extreme tactics.

Extreme Surveillance

While extreme surveillance isn't something the average person needs to be concerned about, professionals employ some interesting tactics to conduct surveillance. Executing these tactics would not be easy for an everyday civilian, as it would require time and resources you just don't have access to. But if your inner spy is curious, there are more complicated means of surveillance that are harder to detect.

Parallel Surveillance

What You'll Need

‣ Two or more vehicles

‣ Knowledge of the roads (they must be parallel)

How it works: The first vehicle would follow the target, keeping a reasonable amount of distance between the cars. The other vehicle would follow the target on streets parallel to the route you are driving on. This enables the additional vehicles to take over the surveillance should the target take a turn.

Leap Frog Surveillance

What You'll Need

‣ Multiple vehicles

‣ Radios

‣ Code words (optional)

How it works: This method requires both multiple vehicles and radios for constant contact. If you really wanted to channel your inner James Bond, you and your partner would create a series of code words to describe what is happening with your target. As the name suggests, this method of surveillance involves telling the people ahead that the target is approaching. This means the original car doesn't need to slow down or pull back, making your presence less obvious to the target.

Try to Confuse the Surveillance Team

The best way to lose someone who may have you under surveillance is to simply start messing with them. Pass a random note
to a complete stranger in order to throw off the surveillance . . .
or walk into a store and start having a random conversation.
These simple actions can confuse or throw off a surveillance
team.

Picket Surveillance

What You'll Need
- A team of individuals
- Radios
- Knowledge of the immediate area

How it works: Executing picket surveillance requires a team
of individuals to be placed at strategic points where your target
may be seen. These individuals would need to be in touch via radio.
If you were using picket surveillance to target someone in New
York City, you would position people at subway entrances, corners,
perhaps a bodega or coffee shop where the target may be likely to
stop. Each individual involved in the surveillance would radio
ahead to alert the others about the position of the target.

It's fun to learn spy tricks and think about how you would ditch
someone if she were following you like how it happens in the movies. It's also empowering to know that you have the capability to

protect yourself should you find yourself in a dangerous situation. Starting today, commit to having an awareness of those around you. Take note of who is in line with you at the store. Pay attention to someone who might be staring at you in a restaurant. Don't discount that car that seems to be taking the exact same route home as you. Acknowledging that these individuals are present—and may be planning to do you harm—is the first step needed to take complete control of your safety. Your commitment to being a confident and aware individual may save your life.

> *Starting today, commit to having an awareness of those around you.*

8

SOCIAL ENGINEERING SECRETS

In a small town in northern England, a young girl and her friends were treated to bumper car rides and ice cream after school by a group of teenage boys. Eventually, these boys went away, and the girls began receiving attention from older men. The free ice cream was replaced by rides in cars, vodka, and marijuana. One young girl started receiving attention from a man twice her age, who appeared to be the leader of his group of men. She told the *New York Times* that he "flattered her" and he eventually bought her drinks and a mobile phone. She liked him. Eventually, after winning her trust, he started raping her. The rapes began gradually, and soon went from weekly to daily. This young victim was then expected to service half a dozen men while locked in the room of an apartment. Unfortunately, this young woman's experience was not unique. It has been estimated that 1,400 children were sexually exploited in Rotherham, England, between 1997 and 2013. The process was the same. Young men would frequent public places like bus stations, shopping malls, and town centers looking for young girls. They would gradually win the girls over with cigarettes and alcohol. Harder drugs were sometimes introduced. One man would begin a sexual relationship with a girl, and he would act as her "boyfriend." The boyfriend would then insist that if the girl really loved him, she would also have sex with other men. At this point, threats and blackmail would be used. One young girl was informed that if she told, her family would be killed. In some cases things got even worse, as some girls were bartered or sold for drugs and guns.

This is a tragic example of how social engineering can be used to manipulate people into doing horrible things they would normally never imagine doing. It seemed innocent enough at first, an ice cream cone from a teenage boy at an arcade—but slowly and gradually a much more sinister plan was revealed, escalating into drugs and alcohol, rides and phones, and eventually exploitation by much older men.

What Is Social Engineering?

At its most basic, social engineering is when a person is psychologically manipulated into taking an action they don't want to take. Social engineering could also involve manipulating someone into giving away confidential information. Social engineering takes many forms, and thankfully, not all of them are as dark. In New York City and other major cities, you can be sitting at a stoplight when a guy comes up to your car and starts spraying your windshield. You'll tell him, "Knock it off. I don't want my windshield cleaned—go away." But he ignores you and just keeps cleaning.

Turns out, he did a great job, and when he comes up to the window you think, "OK, he did clean my windshield, I'll give him two bucks." That window washer has socially engineered you into giving him money. Back in Baltimore, there was a homeless man at the front door of a gas station I used to go to. He'd open the door for me and say "Have a nice day." On the way out he'd open the door for you again, but this time he'd also say "Can you spare a dollar?" I saw lots of people being socially engineered out of dollars by this guy. And is there a single person out there who hasn't received a birthday gift from someone, and thought to yourself, "Now I have to get something for Jim on his birthday." These forms of social engineering are annoying, but not necessarily dangerous. Many criminals, however, have mastered social engineering as a way of getting what they want from innocent people.

While social engineering takes many forms, you may be most familiar with social engineering scams that take place online. For example, many of us have gotten the sob story email from an acquaintance. They're traveling abroad. They've been mugged. They have no passport or credit cards. The embassy is closed, they are completely stranded, and have no other option but to email you out of desperation for your credit card number. Thankfully, most of us recognize this for what it is, a scam. Unfortunately, the scam keeps happening, because there is always someone who is willing to give out a credit card number to help a person in need. It's important to know that social engineering schemes have been happening for centuries, and you're not just vulnerable when you sit down at your computer. From the Trojan Horse to Bernie Madoff's Ponzi scheme, social engineering scams take many forms.

I was once traveling with a friend in France who decided to open up her map the second she got out of the metro. Immediately she was approached by a man offering to help with directions. I knew he was positioning her so that an accomplice working with him could steal her purse. Sure enough, there was another man farther back, waiting to swoop in while the man "helped" give her directions. While this is a classic distraction scam, social engineering scams can get very creative. In New York City, a well-dressed twenty-something man was on his way to meet a colleague when he bumped into a man with a young child. When they collided, a container of Chinese food spilled to the ground. The man carrying the food became incredibly angry. "That's our dinner! You've ruined our dinner! I don't have any more money to feed my kid." While this lifelong New Yorker was suspicious, he still reached into his wallet to get cash for this guy. He knew it was probably a scam, but didn't want to risk a little kid going without dinner. Turns out, scam artists buy the cheapest dish on the menu at a local Chinese takeout joint, bump into a sympathetic looking person, and make a nice profit off of their "ruined dinner." This scam has been updated to include an expensive bottle of wine. Tourists will collide with someone carrying an expensive bottle of wine, be shown a phony receipt to prove it, and asked to fork over $60. The Beijing tea con debuted during the 2008 summer Olympics. Young Chinese girls would befriend a tourist over a period of several hours. At that point, they would suggest that the tourist experience a traditional tea ceremony. The tourist is taken to a teahouse and is not shown a menu. After sampling a small amount of tea during a "traditional ceremony," the tourist is then given a massive bill. Not wanting to appear rude or foolish, the tourist pays the bill in full. It turns out that the girls are working for the proprietor of the teahouse, and he's just managed to turn a hefty profit.

All of these situations involved psychological manipulation—preying on individuals' emotions to entice them to do something they didn't want to do. Fortunately, you can learn to tune in to situations where your decency as a human is being turned against you. The good news is that by understanding some of the underlying causes that allow humans to be scammed and being aware of some common, basic tactics used by criminals, you'll never fall for any of their schemes.

Why We Fall for It: Cognitive Biases

The goal of people executing social engineering techniques is to essentially manipulate us through a crack in our thinking. Con artists are experts at finding human faults and using such weaknesses to do whatever they want. Con artists know how to use a wide range of human emotions in their favor—greed, curiosity, generosity, and fear. While emotions like fear can get us out of trouble, like by telling us to run if we're being chased or to escape if a building is on fire, these feelings can also be used to trap us. What happens in a social engineering scheme is that people fall prey not only to the con artist but to their own cognitive biases as well.

Cognitive biases are basically errors in our thinking that occur while we're trying to process information. Humans need to sort through lots of information, sometimes quickly, to make a decision. Our cognitive biases are a shortcut our brains take to help us get there faster. These shortcuts are extremely helpful in the situations I mentioned previously—when facing danger. Our biases are less helpful when someone is trying to scam us. There are many different kinds of biases that impact our decision making, but if you learn to be aware of just a few key biases, you'll be less likely to fall victim to a scam.

Affect Heuristic

Affect heuristic is what's happening when you're having an immediate gut reaction. It's a fast, instantaneous reaction that uses your emotional responses to help you make a decision. The general idea is that if you feel good about something, you'll assume whatever it is you're feeling good about will have a beneficial impact on your life. Basically, the way you feel colors how you will interpret a particular situation.

What it looks like: If you grew up spending summers having a great time swimming in a lake with your family, the sight of water will have a pleasant, calming effect on you. If you nearly drowned as a child, the sight of water may make you immediately anxious and afraid. Your feelings about water directly impact your reaction to the actual water.

The Decoy Effect

The decoy effect is what happens when you're trying to make a decision between two things and then you discover there's a third option. The third option becomes a way to easily measure the other options against each other. Joe Huber, a marketing professor at Duke University, explained how the decoy effect works by asking a group of people about restaurant preferences. In one scenario, the really great five-star restaurant was a long drive away. The nearby choice was just three stars. The group couldn't decide. Great food and a long ride? Or dinner nearby—but maybe not as good. They felt the five-star would be a no-brainer if it weren't so far away. He introduced a third choice, a two-star restaurant located somewhere between the two other restaurants. This led people to choose the three-star restaurant, because it now beat out the third choice on both location *and* quality.

What it looks like: Not too long ago, we had three simple choices when buying a beverage at a restaurant or a coffee at Dunkin' Donuts or Starbucks—small, medium, and large. With the introduction of super-sizing and tall, many of us, given the additional choice, go for medium when we normally would have gone for small. The decoy effect is causing our brains to weigh the other choices against the new options, and go for the slightly bigger cup.

The Ostrich Effect

People tend to want lots of information, when it's good news. If the information is negative, even if it's helpful, people often opt not to know. As you may have guessed, the ostrich effect refers to a refusal to acknowledge negative information by putting your head in the sand. The general idea is that, "If I can't see it, it doesn't exist."

What it looks like: A typical example of the ostrich effect is not wanting to open your credit card bill after an expensive vacation or a big holiday like Christmas. You know the information is likely to make you unhappy, so you simply don't open the bill until you absolutely have to. You're avoiding any potentially negative feelings by not letting yourself have access to the information.

Optimism Bias

While humans need to feel hopeful to make progress, we have a tendency to be more optimistic than *realistic*. People tend to expect things to turn out much better than they actually do. This tendency to see our future in a positive light means we aren't preparing for potential dangers and are left vulnerable.

What it looks like: A person who is overly optimistic about the future may not be able to prepare for some life events that are, in fact, entirely possible. Such a person may not save money to have a cushion in the event of a job loss. Or an overly optimistic viewpoint may make that trip to the doctor for an annual physical seem unnecessary. Not saving money or seeing medical professionals on a regular basis can of course have very negative if not disastrous results.

Recency Bias

Recency bias is our tendency to think that what's happening lately—any trends or patterns that we see now—is likely to continue into the future. It's easier for humans to remember the impact of recent events. So rather than relying on actual data or realizing that there are some events that can't be predicted, we go ahead with the assumption that life will continue along similar lines.

What it looks like: Recency bias could mean not taking a hurricane warning seriously and refusing to take appropriate measures because your area has never seen a hurricane before.

Don't Let Cognitive Biases Get You Scammed

While there are even more cognitive biases than the common ones I've just described, there are a few things you can do to make sure cognitive biases won't get you scammed. Having a healthy sense of skepticism can keep you safe. I'm not saying you need to be worried 24/7 about getting scammed, but be aware. If someone asks to help you read a map in a foreign country, take a minute to look over your shoulder and make sure you're safe. If someone shows up at your door saying they're the police, you need to call 911 to verify that it's true. Be cautious and don't be afraid to check your surroundings or verify information to ensure your safety.

There's a Scam Born Every Minute

We've all heard the phrase "There's a sucker born every minute." The truth is, there are new scams born every minute, especially in the Internet age. While I couldn't possible list every scam that's been played, I can make you aware of some of the most prevalent scams out there. By familiarizing yourself with some of the most common scamming techniques, you'll be ready to immediately avoid the situation should someone try to pull one off on you.

The Law of Reciprocity: When You Don't Necessarily Want to Return the Favor

We've all been in a situation where we genuinely want to return a favor. If a neighbor takes in your mail while you're on vacation, or a family member babysits your kid while you're in a pinch—it's normal to want to pay them back by lending a helpful hand. Essentially if someone does something nice for us, we have a natural inclination to return the favor. In some instances, however, our natural inclination to return favors can get us in big trouble. This is the case when someone purposefully exploits the law of reciprocity and expects something much bigger than she's given in return. For example, your neighbor may have agreed to walk your dog on a day when you were away, which is a nice thing to do. You'd likely be comfortable doing something similar in return, like feeding her cat or watering her plants while she's on vacation. It wouldn't make sense however, if she showed up one day and let you know she expected you to paint her house or mow her lawn for the entire summer. The trouble starts when criminals use the law of reciprocity against someone by expecting much larger things than they've given in return.

On May 1, 1990, Pamela Ann Smart came home from work to find her home ransacked and her husband shot dead. After a sensational trial, Smart was convicted for conspiring in a first-degree murder that was ultimately carried out by her fifteen-year-old lover and two of his friends. Smart met the teen, William Flynn, at a school program where they both were volunteers. As their relationship developed, she confided in Flynn that she'd like to see her husband dead. Eventually Smart threatened to stop having sex with Flynn unless he agreed to kill her husband. Flynn was sentenced to twenty-eight years to life for his involvement in this murder. The other teens were convicted of murder conspiracy or accomplice charges. During the trial, it came out that Smart had accused Flynn of not loving her. She told him if he really loved her, he would be willing to kill her husband.

Smart used the law of reciprocity against Flynn to get what she wanted. She initiated a relationship with a vulnerable young person, gave this person sex, and insisted that something was to be done for her in return. Obviously this is not how normal relationships work—Smart set up a situation that allowed her to socially engineer someone into committing murder for her. In the intelligence world, the law of reciprocity may start with someone buying drinks for you . . . or gifts, and then asking for a small favor. This small favor usually represents the beginning of a very slippery slope. The bottom line is, even if you owe someone a favor, you should by no means feel guilted into doing something that doesn't feel right to you.

Why You Don't Always Want to Be the Good Samaritan

Tymikia Jackson was pumping gas in a Georgia gas station when she was approached by a couple looking for help. A woman asked her if she would give her some money to put gas in her car. Jackson wanted to help the couple and happily handed over the last $20 bill she had in her wallet. The woman thanked Jackson and was so happy that she asked if she could have a hug. Jackson complied. A man got out of the driver's seat and approached Jackson. He said, "Thank you so much. I really appreciate it. Can I please have a hug?" Jackson noted that the hug felt different. The next morning, Jackson figured out why the couple were anxious to give her a hug: about $3,000 was missing from her bank account. Only a couple of hours after she left the gas station there were two large charges on her debit card and withdrawals from ATMs. It turns out that while they were hugging her, the thieves used high-tech scanning devices to take information from her credit cards, which were in her front pocket.

Jackson is actually lucky it was just her credit card number that was taken. Putting yourself at someone's mercy as a Good Samaritan can cost you your life. While it's admirable to want to help others—especially those in desperate need—it's essential that by doing so you don't put yourself in a position where you could be harmed.

Ted Bundy, the notorious serial killer who confessed to thirty homicides committed in seven different states in the 1970s, was a master of the Good Samaritan scam. Bundy was known for being handsome and very charismatic. He tended to approach his potential victims posing as an injured person. It was not unusual for him to use crutches, and plaster of Paris for making casts was found in one of his homes. When women were disappearing at a college campus about sixty miles southeast of Seattle, several witnesses reported seeing a man fitting his description—with his leg in a cast, or his arm in a sling—asking for help carrying things to his car.

Obviously not everyone asking for help is in fact a depraved serial killer. However, Bundy's story illustrates how easy it is to become vulnerable when agreeing to do something as simple as help an injured person walk a few feet to their car. It is our instinct as human beings to do good, but it's important to not let a desire to be a helpful person reign over safety. In Batesville, Indiana, a man pretended to be a stranded motorist, looking for Good Samaritans to scam. He'd pull over to the side of the interstate and wait for help to come along. When an elderly woman stopped, he was able to convince her to lend him money so that he could repair a mechanical problem with his vehicle. The con artist then called the same Good Samaritan the next day. Unfortunately, she still didn't recognize the scam, and she gave the man directions to her house so that he could pay her back. When he arrived at the residence, he entered the home without permission and distracted the woman long enough to steal her wallet. In Vancouver, Shirley Magliocco was returning from a trip to the grocery store. A couple approached her in her driveway, asking her for water for their overheated van. When she walked into the house, she forgot to turn off her alarm system, and went upstairs to turn it off. As soon as she came downstairs the couple was gone, and so was her wallet.

The bottom line is that there are countless ways a criminal can take advantage of your good nature. Before agreeing to assist someone, make sure you're not isolating yourself, don't ever get in someone's vehicle, and don't be afraid to leave immediately or call for help if you're uncomfortable.

Pretexting

In *Die Hard 4: Live Free or Die*, the character Matt Farrell (played by Justin Long) successfully uses a fake illness as a pretext. He tells the OnStar assist representative that he needs the car to get to his father who is dying of a heart attack. This convinces the representative to start the car, which Farrell is actually in the process of stealing.

Pretexting is when a scenario is invented to engage a person so that he will perform actions or give away information that he wouldn't be willing to do otherwise. Pretexting often involves an elaborate lie. A criminal engaging in pretexting may impersonate coworkers, a bank employee, an insurance investigator, tax authorities, or even a clergyman. A pretexter may impersonate any person who could be perceived as having the power to get a person into a particular situation or who has the right to know certain information.

In Manatee, Florida, a woman might owe her life to successfully recognizing a pretext. Late on a Sunday night, a woman pulled over after she saw red and green flashing lights. A tall, clean-shaven male asked her to get into his vehicle. He did not ask for license and registration, so she refused to get out of her car. The man told her he was going back to his car to call for a female officer, but instead fled the scene at a high speed. This woman would not normally have gotten into a car with a stranger. Luckily she had the awareness to recognize that the situation was engineered to get her into his vehicle. After the car pulled off she immediately called 911.

How Can You Spot a Pretext?

- The pretexter usually prepares by having answers ready. He anticipates what he may need to know to sound authoritative. A good pretexter is quick and ready to handle whatever direction the situation may go. Trust your gut and know something might be off if the person doesn't have all the answers. An example of this is the guy who pulls a woman over but isn't wearing a uniform or driving a marked car.
- The details don't add up. Imagine a friend telling you, "Oh, we're just having a small family dinner for New Year's." Yet there are thirty cars parked in front of her house and you can hear the music from all the way down the street.
- It's too good to be true. Not many of us have wealthy Nigerian uncles. If you get an email saying he has $50 million waiting for you, it's a scam and you should ignore it.

‣ Your credit card company shouldn't be calling you, asking for personal information. If your credit card company calls you, hang up and call them using the number on the back of your card.

Distraction Robberies

There's a man in Tennessee who is probably very regretful that he let himself be the victim of a distraction robbery. Stephen Amaral from Crossville, Tennessee, was approached by a couple with a very unusual request. A woman asked Amaral if she could "take a skinny dip in his pool" while her husband went out to buy cigarettes. Amaral proceeded to watch the woman swim naked in his pool for about twenty minutes. Turns out, while Amaral was watching her swim and even providing her with a towel, her husband was inside robbing his house.

People are easily distracted, and criminals know this. It's not terribly difficult to choose a person, or even a group, and create a means of distraction. At times the distraction may be high impact. In Grenada, Mississippi, three people were arrested after calling in bomb threats to two area schools. While the police were searching and evacuating the campuses of the two schools, two masked men robbed a local bank. Most distractions, however, are going to be smaller scale, and the criminal will attempt to distract you immediately and quickly. The criminal hopes you won't suspect a thing—until you realize your purse or wallet is missing. In San Clemente, California, an eighty-six-year-old man lost $200,000 worth of jewelry. A man approached the elderly homeowner posing as a contractor. He offered his roofing services, which the man accepted. The man was told that the contractor's son was with him. He asked the elderly man to watch out for him while he went up on the roof. Meanwhile, the "contractor" entered the house and stole jewelry. On High Street in London, a woman withdrew a large amount of cash before heading to the grocery store. She was approached by a group of two men and a woman, who told her she had "something on her back." They insisted on helping her wipe it off. While she was distracted, the cash disappeared from her handbag. While many criminals choose to target the elderly when pulling off a distraction robbery, anyone can be a victim to this type of crime.

Like the Good Samaritan scam, distraction scams can get pretty imaginative. There are no limits to what a criminal will do to distract you. So how do you avoid becoming the victim of a distraction?

- **Keep your distance.** If something seems odd, stay back and do not let the person get close to you. This prevents the person from picking your pocket or from attacking you, should that be their intent.
- **Look behind you.** I once walked out of my local grocery store when a woman approached me and asked me for a ride. This is clearly not typical behavior, so I quickly looked around to make sure someone wasn't coming to hit me over the head and rob me.
- **Ask questions.** Ask more questions about the person's story, and make sure it adds up. Don't take what someone tells you at face value. If she's trying to distract you, she won't be able to answer all of your questions—she'll go away when you start questioning her.

Your Inner Spy: How to Social Engineer Someone into Doing What You Want Them to Do

You wouldn't think so, but CIA officers are often the target of social engineering. It's not uncommon for CIA officers to be approached in a bar, often by a beautiful woman with a big story to tell. CIA officers are even warned about being pitched out in public. I remember I was once in a bar with some of the other officers after work, and I was approached by a woman, who I quickly learned was from Belarus. I didn't know this woman at all, but that didn't stop her from launching into an incredible story about her life. She told me that she was terribly abused by her brute of a husband—she had been sold to this forty-something guy when she was only eighteen. She eventually got away from him and into a shelter, where she suffered even more abuse. Despite all of this, she somehow managed to get out of these terrible situations and put herself through medical school. Her willingness to open up and share such personal and tragic information was a red flag for me. I knew she was expecting me to open up with just as much information in return—and who knows who she was going to give it to? Luckily, because of my training, I wasn't going to reciprocate by giving out equally personal information. This woman also was not exhibiting normal human behavior. If someone wants to hit on you at a bar, they're going to put their best foot forward, not open up with a story about being a mail-order bride who was raped by her husband.

How Social Engineering Can Work for You

While I'm certainly not suggesting that you use social engineering to do anyone harm, I will admit that it's possible to have some fun with it. There are plenty of ways we convince others to do things we'd like them to do. Following are a few of the more imaginative ways you could use social engineering to your advantage—and techniques you should keep in mind in order to avoid being socially engineered yourself.

Hire a Bodyguard

Have you ever wondered what it feels like to be famous? Twenty-three-year-old Brett Cohen used social engineering to find out. After checking out Times Square in New York City, Cohen decided it was the perfect place to make his debut as a celebrity. Cohen created his own entourage, hiring two bodyguards off of Craigslist, three cameramen and four photographers. Cohen, who is a regular-looking guy, put on a nice shirt, a pair of dark glasses and a bright smile. Cohen carefully exited the 30 Rock building in Rockefeller Center, flanked by two large and serious looking security guards. His cameramen and photographers got right to work. Cohen flashed a huge grin, and exuded confidence. He blew kisses into the crowd. The crowd ate it up immediately. Cohen had a friend ask people what they thought about the famous Brett Cohen. One man said he was "a very good actor," referring to a part he obviously did not play in a Spider-Man movie. Another man was asked what he thought of Cohen's music. The man replied that he had "heard his first single." Cohen posed for pictures with fans as they followed him around Times Square for three hours. A group of girls, who were screaming and blowing kisses, said, "This is the best day of my life! I love him! He's beautiful." Toward the end of the prank Cohen had nearly three hundred people following him. Concerned the police would get involved because of the large crowd that was gathering, Cohen had his two security guards escort him into a small hotel, gesturing to the crowds to stay back. In the video he made of the experience, Cohen is seen after it's all over, walking down the street, and onto the subway alone. Once his entourage was gone, so apparently was his celebrity.

Borrow a Baby

If you want people to put their guard down, chances are, having a baby with you will help. I'll admit that this one is most likely going to work only for a man. Unfortunately, we're brainwashed, and the truth is, we don't think twice about a woman taking care of a baby. If a father takes the baby out to the grocery store? He's automatically considered father of the year. A friend of mine noted that her husband got a completely different reaction from nurses at the pediatrician's office than she would have. Her husband took their sick baby in to see the doctor, and left the diaper bag at home. The baby got hungry and started wailing for food. The nurses immediately jumped in with a bottle and formula and were basically just impressed that dad was taking the baby to the doctor at all. "If it were me, and I had forgotten the bottle, I would have been viewed as the worst mother ever. But my husband gets praised just for showing up!" If a man is holding a baby out in public and asks for help, chances are most people will be eager and quick to respond to a helpless father. There's something about the presence of babies and children that just make people more comfortable. We've all heard stories about the guy who takes his nephew out to the park to play baseball but just happens to pick up a woman in the process.

Quid Pro Quo

Anyone who has seen *The Silence of the Lambs* probably remembers the scene where Jodi Foster is trying to get information about a serial killer she's pursuing, from another serial killer, Hannibal Lecter (played by Anthony Hopkins).

> *If I help you, Clarice, it will be "turns" for us too. Quid pro quo—I tell you things, you tell me things. Not about this case, though. About yourself. Quid pro quo. Yes or no?*

Quid pro quo simply means "something for something." A classic example of quid pro quo behavior is the guy who takes a woman out for a fancy dinner and expects her to come home with him. Quid pro quo tactics can easily be used in less ominous ways. A wife who wants her husband to do something around the house might make his favorite dinner before asking him. A teenager might go ahead and clean out the garage, hoping that in return he'll be allowed to stay out late or borrow the car. Most of us use quid pro quo tactics without even realizing it. It's an easy way to get someone to do a much-needed favor, and this is essentially another example of the law of reciprocity in action.

Act like You're Supposed to Be There

In the movie *Wedding Crashers*, Jeremy (played by Vince Vaughn) and his buddy John (Owen Wilson) are able to crash just about any wedding, even the wedding of the year: that of the secretary of state's daughter. They boldly walk in, introduce themselves, have a glass of Champagne, and have no trouble making up a bogus reason about how they got invited. Acting like you're supposed to be there is a powerful way to gain access to a place you're not supposed to be. I'm not suggesting you show up where you're not wanted or do anything illegal, but it's fun to take a look at how some people manage to pull this off. I've easily gotten into buildings for building penetration jobs because I chatted up the security guard and acted like I was supposed to be there. Society is brainwashed to believe in the power of a badge or ID. People see a company ID, even one easily made at home, and assume immediately you're on the up and up.

People who manage to gain access to venues and parties have mastered a few key skills. They appear completely comfortable and confident, even though they may actually be sweating inside. They've probably taken the time to make sure they blend effortlessly into the environment they are infiltrating. For example, had Owen Wilson's character shown up to the secretary of state's wedding in a bad suit, he might have stuck out. Gaining access to places you're not supposed to be means appearing like you have control of your surroundings. Don't look around checking the place out; you need to move around naturally, like you've been there many times before.

Find Their Motivation

Everyone has a motivation—something that drives him. We all have different interests and hobbies that make us unique individuals. But if we're not careful, our motivations can be used against us. I enjoy shooting and really like guns, and it's pretty easy to find this information about me. I wouldn't let someone's shared interest in guns lure me into an off-the-beaten path gun store where he could do me harm. But sometimes finding others' motivations is a good way to socially engineer them.

I heard a story about a few men hitting on a beautiful model at

**I'm Worried That My Elderly Parents Will
Become Victims of Scam Artists. What Can I Do
to Prevent Them from Becoming Victims?**

It's true that the elderly are often the targets for scams. Have a
conversation with your parents, and make it clear that no one
from their bank or credit card companies will ever call them or
email them asking for their password or account number. If that
happens, they should call the bank (looking up the number for
the bank themselves). This is a common problem, as the elderly
tend to be trustworthy. I simply tell my dad that if he ever has a
second of doubt, he should call me immediately and we'll talk
about it.

a bar. The first guy was a billionaire businessman. He approached
the woman and was immediately shot down. The second guy was
a famous movie producer. He didn't do any better than the mil-
lionaire. The third guy was fat and short. The other guys see him
whisper into this woman's ear, and before the other men know it
the couple is leaving together. The couple return to the bar an hour
later and go their separate ways. The businessman has to know.
He walks up to the short guy and says, "What did you say to her?"
The short guy tells him, "I asked her if she'd like to come back to
my place and do cocaine." The third guy found her motivation.

Obviously it wasn't too hard to find this woman's motivation.
It's important that you take steps to make sure someone can't easily
find out what motivates you. Those of you who use Facebook, make

sure you use privacy settings and be careful about what "friends" can learn about you from visiting your page. If it's obvious you're a graduate of a particular college, work in a certain industry, and enjoy hiking—it would be easy enough for someone to get in your good graces by sharing those common interests. I'm not suggesting everyone you meet who has a shared interest with you has dark intentions—just think twice about letting your guard down because a guy you meet at a bar likes the same bands and also volunteers with children.

9

HOW TO BE A HUMAN LIE DETECTOR

It's a long process to get hired as a CIA Officer. It can take over a year to complete the psychological exam, physical exam, background checks, paperwork, and various interviews. One of the most nerve-racking parts of the experience for me was the polygraph test. I was actually offered jobs by both the Secret Service and the CIA, so I've been polygraphed multiple times. When you're taking a polygraph test, sensors are attached to different parts of your body to measure your respiratory rate, blood pressure, heart rate, and electrodermal activity (in other words, how much you sweat). While I was obviously aware of what all the wires were for, I couldn't see anything that was happening with the polygraph machine. During my polygraph for the Secret Service, I remember being in a tiny white room with no windows. The white walls almost had a hypnotizing effect. The chair was uncomfortable, and I was seated just a couple of feet away from the guy who was conducting the test. I was hooked up to several wires. I remember thinking about a story from my family's past, and was nervous about how it would impact my polygraph test.

One summer, when I was about nine years old, I found an interesting poster when we were cleaning out my grandmother's basement. I thought it was really neat; it was colorful and had a Russian hammer and sickle on it.

I wanted to keep it, but my mom said that there was no way my dad would let me put it in my bedroom. Turns out, my grandmother was a full-blown communist (not a phrase many people toss around these days), and this poster was communist propaganda. It seems my grandmother's brother, who had gone to Russia several times, had convinced her to join the Communist Party. My dad was even dragged to her communist book club meetings when he was a kid. To make the story more interesting, my dad's piano teacher at that time was an undercover FBI agent. My grandfather, who was a farmer, often had FBI agents come out to question him, even though he did not share my grandmother's communist views. Luckily for her, they didn't deem my grandmother a threat to national security. Obviously, my family's former communist ties were a bit of a concern for me when I was applying to work for the Secret Service. When I was asked, "Have you had any foreign affiliation with foreign governments, or worked with the Russian government?" I ended up just laughing, and telling the truth.

Luckily, that's not the first question they asked me. The first thing that happens when you take a polygraph test is that a baseline is established. As you know from learning about situational awareness, a baseline is a measure of what's normal for you. To take a baseline measurement during a polygraph test, you'll be asked a series of simple questions that you obviously know the answer to: "What's your name?" "Where do you live?" Once they can see your reaction to simple questions, they'll start to ask more challenging ones.

When I took my polygraph for the CIA, the polygraphers actually did a kind of good cop–bad cop routine when they got to the tougher questions. I have never done drugs in my life, so when one officer was asked if I've ever taken drugs, I answered no. Yet the other officer was saying to me "The polygraph is showing that you've done drugs. You're lying. We realize everyone has done drugs in high school or college." It was a ploy to get a person to admit they had done drugs after pushing them to the limit. Luckily, I had the sense to stick with the truth. In the scheme of things, my polygraph turned out to be easy. I know other officers who were told to come back the next day for a follow-up. I was in and out in just a couple of hours. I was relieved when the experience was over.

One of the best benefits of working in the intelligence business is that you basically become a human lie detector. I probably don't need to tell you why this is an incredibly useful skill. We all want to be able to trust our business associates, employees, neighbors, friends, and the people who interact with our children. We may be working with a contractor or in the middle of an important business negotiation when something in our gut is telling us not to believe what this person is saying. How do we know if we should trust our gut if we think someone is being truthful? Luckily, there are some simple tricks you can train yourself to look out for that will help you determine whether a person is lying.

Human beings are terrible liars. This is the way we are wired. Our brains move a million miles a second, and before we can think straight enough to tell a lie we've already given off many subtle clues that we're not telling the truth.

And while a person telling a lie will not necessarily exhibit all of the traits I'm going to talk about in this chapter, it's important to learn to notice them when they come up. A person who exhibits a cluster of these behaviors is likely telling a lie.

A situation I found myself in my sophomore year of high school provides a good example of some of the classic traits exhibited by a liar. I was dating a girl who had just broken up with a defensive linebacker from the high school football team. This guy was intense, and wasn't going to appreciate me dating his ex-girlfriend. It's important to note that at the time, I was scrawny (not that I'm a giant by any means now). This guy could have easily taken me in a fight. One afternoon I was at her house when the ex-boyfriend pulled up in his car. The girlfriend didn't know what to do. She panicked and told me to go hide in one of the closets. She let the linebacker in, and he immediately wanted to know what was going on. She told him no one was there, but that didn't stop him from opening and closing all the doors in the house. I was cowering in the back of her closet when he opened the door. I was sure that was going to be the end of me. He saw me and said, "Oh, hi Jason. What are you doing here?" When trying to detect a lie, the first three to five seconds of a confrontation are crucial—that's the time when our brains are working frantically to try to keep up with the lie we're trying to tell. When the guy first asked me what I was doing, I was stuttering. A few seconds later I said, "There's a girl I like in school. I came over to get advice. I'm hiding, because I'm embarrassed and I don't want anyone to know . . . so don't tell anyone." I was rambling like crazy, because I was lying and my mind was work-

> **Human beings are terrible liars.**

ing to create the lie. (In case you're wondering, the linebacker believed me.)

The story of my sophomore year girlfriend outlines a couple of typical lying behaviors that indicate that someone is not telling the truth. I stumbled in the first few seconds of the confrontation because I had to come up with the lie. If I were telling the truth and had nothing to hide, I wouldn't have stuttered or been delayed with my response—I would have immediately given an answer. While I'm lucky the linebacker was willing to believe my ridiculous story, if he had known just a few of the basic signs about lying, I would have been in big trouble.

Establish a Baseline

While it would be great to jump right in and give you a list of behaviors to look out for to determine if someone is lying, the thing is, that won't work if you don't take the time to establish a baseline. The CIA or any other intelligence agency doesn't sit you down in a chair, strap some wires to you, and jump in with big questions like "Have you ever used drugs?" or "Have you ever worked for a foreign government?" Instead, as I noted earlier, they need to establish a baseline by asking you basic questions about yourself and maybe even something as simple as, "Is the carpet in this room green?" Once the CIA could see my breathing rate, pulse, blood pressure, and perspiration rate when I answered those simple questions in an obviously truthful way, they knew what my baseline was. They'd now be able to determine more easily if I was lying when answering other, more difficult questions.

What's the Person's Baseline?

To really establish whether someone is lying to you or not, you need to get yourself familiar with their everyday, regular behavior. If you don't know what constitutes normal behavior for this person, you won't have a clue if they are exhibiting some of the signs that indicate a lie is being told. If you decide a person is lying about accidentally scratching your car in a parking lot because she is "acting fidgety," you could be completely wrong. That person may be fidgety all the time, and you couldn't have possibly have established a baseline in the ten seconds since you first met her. However, baseline behavior can be established fairly quickly and easily using the following tactics.

Tactic One: Make Him Comfortable

While movies and TV shows are full of scenes where a cop or a criminal is practically torturing someone to get an answer out of him, in real life, it's best to make sure the person you're trying to get a baseline from is comfortable. I would make sure we were sitting on a couch and would ask him if he wants a drink of water. You're more liable to get an accurate read of his baseline behavior this way. On the flip side, if it's a hundred degrees outside and both of us are sweating bullets, I wouldn't try to figure out if a person was lying under those uncomfortable conditions. If I knew the person well enough to know if he had certain phobias, I'd avoid those too. I wouldn't try to figure out if he is lying while at the top of the Empire State Building if I knew he was afraid of heights—and I wouldn't have my dog nearby if I knew the person was afraid of dogs.

Tactic Two: Ask What He Already Knows

When trying to establish a person's baseline behavior I'll ask him questions he already knows the answer to. Think of simple questions that the person has no reason to lie about. For example, you might know that your coworker used to work at Macy's. Simply ask him, "So you worked at Macy's? How was that job?" Because he has no reason to lie when answering a simple question like this, you'll get some good clues about how the person behaves when telling the truth.

Tactic Three: Watch Him Like a Hawk

While he's answering these innocuous questions, you need to watch your subject closely in order to note any unusual mannerisms or behaviors. Make a mental note of anything he does while answering, which establishes a baseline. You need to observe and note every mannerism the person exhibits during tactics one and two. Here are just a few examples of basic mannerisms:

- Tapping a foot
- Tossing hair
- Biting fingernails
- Unusual facial expressions
- Lowering the eyes
- Sighing
- Throat clearing
- Playing with clothes (adjusting tie, collar, sleeves, etc.)

If you are able to note which mannerisms a person exhibits while *not* lying, it will be much easier to note any changes in behavior that suggest a lie.

The Lying Behaviors

Now that you've spent some time observing your subject and have a grasp of his baseline behaviors, you're ready to start asking questions that relate directly to the lie you suspect you've been told. It is important to note that a person who is lying is not likely to exhibit every behavior I'm going to discuss in this chapter. If a person shows one trait on this list, it does not mean he is lying. What you need to look for are groups of behavior. Is the person exhibiting a few of these signs? If a grouping of these behaviors is present, and you've noted that these behaviors are not part of the person's baseline, it's likely he is telling a lie.

The First Three to Five Seconds

As I mentioned, if a person is lying to you, he will likely exhibit some telltale behaviors within three to five seconds of being asked a question that pertains to the lie. The person may start stuttering or won't be able to get his story out precisely. He may stumble over details as he is trying to answer your question. This happens as our brains take the time to create the lie we actually end up telling. If you ask an employee, "Do you know who took the money from the cash register?" it's crucial you pay close attention to how the person reacts in that three-to-five-second window.

The Indirect Answer

A guilty person will not answer your questions directly.

A guilty person will start listing all the reasons why you should trust him. He'll start to tell you about all the wonderful things he's done. You may hear about how he was an Eagle Scout . . . or how he volunteers with the homeless. While being an Eagle Scout or a volunteer is wonderful, it's no replacement for the truth. An honest person will simply answer your question, rather than try to convince you of his honesty by telling you about all of his good deeds.

Religion

Much like being an Eagle Scout doesn't mean you're honest, being religious doesn't automatically make you trustworthy either. It's not unusual for a person who is lying to try to convince you he can be trusted based on religious beliefs. After getting a deal with Daymond John on the ABC television show *Shark Tank*, I was approached by many people about various deals. In one case, I asked an individual to show me some numbers about a potential deal we were discussing. Instead of showing me what I asked for, he kept saying "Jason, I'm a Christian. You can trust me." This was a red flag. If he were honest, he simply would have sent me what I asked for.

As previously mentioned, I'm Mormon. When I got the deal on *Shark Tank*, John wanted to see my tax returns and my books to make sure the numbers I gave him about my business were accurate. If I had told him, "Daymond, I'm Mormon, you don't need to see my books. You can trust me," that would have been crazy. I don't care what your religion is. If a potential partner asks to see your books and you're an honest person, the only answer should be, "Absolutely."

The Feet

Many people think that we'll be able to catch a person in a lie by watching her face—that a sudden facial expression, a movement of the mouth or eyes is going to provide a sure giveaway that she's lying. The truth is, our feet give away more information than our faces do. If you are sitting at a table or on a sofa with someone, and her feet start jiggling when you ask her a potentially damaging question, it's possible she's lying. In other words, if her feet are still, but then you ask her a question about missing money, and her feet start shifting or jiggling, there's a good chance she's lying. Feet can give you clues in other situations too. Our feet naturally point us in the direction they want to go. For example, if you're talking to someone at a party, and his feet are pointed toward a door, there's a good chance that on some level, he is thinking about getting away. Customs agents are trained to watch people's feet. An honest person who is going through customs at the airport is going to face the customs agent with his feet pointing directly at the person. Honest people don't feel guilty or look like they have some-

> *Our feet give away more information than our faces do.*

thing to hide. If a person is talking to a customs agent, but his feet are not squared up with the agent, the agent knows there's a possibility that the person is lying. A drug smuggler, or a person who has something else to hide is going to have his feet pointed toward the nearest exit when going through customs.

The Freeze

Think of the freeze as a movement that's like a tortoise retreating into its shell. It's common for a person who is guilty to move around less and freeze. This is one of the biggest indicators you're going to get that someone is telling a lie. I fly a lot, and one time I started to notice a very nasty smell. Someone on the plane had obviously passed some gas. I start looking around . . . like where in the world did *that* come from? I notice everyone else is looking around wondering the exact same thing, except for a guy in the row ahead of me on the left. He's sitting there, frozen, while everyone else is looking around (which is what normal people do). This guy was not moving at all, and it was obvious that he was the culprit.

The Over-Stare

Eyes can certainly provide clues that a person is lying, but not necessarily for the reasons you might think. Many people believe that a person who is lying will look down—but there are many other reasons why a person may be looking down. If you just started a new job, and the CEO of the company asked you into the office to question you about missing files from his desk, chances are you'd look down automatically due to the gap in authority. It's an intimidating situation and it's natural to look down. However, if the person is lying she would be more likely to stare too hard at the person questioning her. The over-stare is used when a liar is trying to convince you she's being honest by looking at you directly and intensely—trying too hard to convince you of the truth and simply not exhibiting normal human behavior.

One time, when I was still in the CIA, I was traveling overseas on a personal vacation. When you travel for pleasure or personal reasons as a CIA officer, you definitely don't say you work for the CIA when going through customs in a foreign country. When I got to the customs counter, the agent started grilling me hard. He was asking me a ton of questions. I had my story planned. When she asked me about my job, I told her that I "work at museums in the Washington, DC, area. I do security work, giving people directions and helping them find their way around." While I was telling my story to the customs officer, I was forcing myself not to stare too hard and to break my gaze at her. I made sure to look down occasionally, so the customs agent wouldn't get suspicious about what I was telling her. (It worked.)

The Overreaction

People who are lying tend to have extreme overreactions when confronted. Their intention is to beat you down—and make you feel ridiculous for even questioning their behavior. By overreacting, they're setting up a scenario in which you'll never want to question them again. For example, it's not uncommon for me to be asked about cheating husbands. I was once asked by a woman who found some incriminating evidence on her husband's phone how she could find out if he was having an affair. She insisted he couldn't be having an affair, since their marriage was in great shape. I suggested she confront her husband, tell him about the evidence she found, and see how he reacts. She called me the next day, thrilled that her husband wasn't having an affair. She explained that he was outraged by her suggestion and was extremely upset by the idea that she didn't trust him. Unfortunately, this was actually a big red flag. If you're married and aren't cheating on your wife, and she accuses you of having an affair, chances are that you're not going to fly off the handle. If the truth is you're not cheating, then you ultimately have no reason to be so angry that you're cussing and shouting and completely losing your cool. This woman eventually received definitive proof that her husband was having an affair, and to this day she's amazed that I knew. So the next time someone reacts in a crazy manner when you ask him a question, remember that this is an indicator that he could be lying.

The Light Punisher

It's no surprise that someone who is guilty is going to be more inclined to suggest a lighter punishment. That's why it can be effective to ask the guilty party what *she* thinks the punishment should be. The innocent people involved may suggest appropriate or particularly harsh punishments for the wrongdoer. They might feel a person who steals at work should be fired or arrested and sent to jail. I recently was told about a situation in which someone had broken into a restaurant and had taken $4,000. While trying to figure out what happened, the police gave questionnaires to all of the employees that included questions about what should happen to the person who stole the $4,000. A long-term employee wrote something along the lines of "People make mistakes. They should be told to never do it again." Aware that this was a sign of guilt, the police confronted the person, who eventually confessed.

The Indirect Answer

Liars will often not answer your question directly. Wanting to deflect their guilt, they'll do anything to avoid answering the question. My two-year-old daughter loves her Cabbage Patch doll, but my wife doesn't like her to have it at bedtime. My daughter plays with it, and it keeps her from falling asleep. One night, my daughter was happily playing with her doll, but I knew I had to take it away from her before bed. The second I took it she started yelling and screaming. So what did I do? I gave it back because I was exhausted after a long day and I wanted to go to sleep. My wife, immediately suspicious, asked me if I gave her the doll back. Instead of answering yes, I immediately asked, "What?" My indirect answer was a strong indication that I was lying and had given the doll back to my screaming daughter (but I happened to be joking when answering my wife's question, and she knew it). If someone you suspect of lying answers with another question or simply refuses to answer at all, this is another indication that she might be guilty of lying.

The Head Shake

While this may be more difficult to detect, watching how a person shakes his head can be an indicator of lying. In short, if you ask a person a question, and he answers honestly, his head moves before the words come out of his mouth.

If his head shakes yes or no after he has already started speaking, chances are he's telling a lie. In her popular TED talk "How to Spot a Liar," Pamela Meyer illustrates this point by showing an interview with former presidential candidate John Edwards. The interview was about fathering a child with a woman he was having an affair with. While Edwards was emphatically telling the interviewer that he'd be happy to take a paternity test, Meyers shows us that Edwards was very subtly shaking his head in the negative during the entire interview. The words coming out of his mouth were in direct conflict with his head movement. While difficult to see, this is a sign that Edwards was not being honest.

10

HOW TO DISAPPEAR WITHOUT A TRACE

Michelle Kramer was concerned when she woke up to discover that her husband wasn't home. She had hoped that Mark, a successful surgeon in the Chicago area, had simply gone out for a run. Michelle had noted that her husband hadn't been himself lately. He had been stressed out about some malpractice lawsuits. Mark had even asked her if she would be willing to move to Europe to live a "simpler life," which is why they were living on a yacht in Greece when he went missing. When Mark didn't return to the boat, Michelle started to suspect that he had disappeared on purpose. After a whirlwind romance, Mark and Michelle lived a lavish lifestyle. They took private jets to vacations in Greece and Italy. When Michelle eventually made it back home, she found her elaborate lifestyle had disappeared along with her husband. She discovered there was no money left in their bank accounts, and that he had been performing surgeries on patients in volume, to make fast cash. There had been more than three hundred malpractice suits filed against him, and they were $6 million in debt. Another five years passed before Mark was found—in a tent on top of Mont Blanc, the highest mountain in the Alps, with canned food, clothing, and other survival gear. He was caught when he failed to pay rent on an apartment he sometimes stayed in in a nearby Italian town. Strangely enough, he used his real name to rent the apartment, and when he didn't pay rent, his landlord went to the police. While Mark Kramer chose to disappear rather than deal with the many problems he'd created, there are unfortunately times when innocent people feel they have no choice but to disappear off the face of the earth. With some extra careful planning and commitment to carrying out that plan, it is possible to vanish and not be found. I'm certainly not suggesting you try this yourself, but I'm often asked how it's done. Here's how.

The Basics

While possible, disappearing is complicated, stressful, and requires meticulous planning. If you truly believed the only way to stay alive is to be gone forever, you would to have to stay off the grid long term, which is mentally taxing as well as logistically challenging. That's why I consider disappearing truly a last resort. If restraining orders, police protection, legal help, and other such avenues haven't produced satisfactory results, disappearing may be the right option for you—but chances are, this information is more of a "who knew?" than a "try this at home." It goes without saying that anyone even casually considering this route should think carefully before taking action. Consider the following:

Resources: If you were to disappear, you would need access to lots of cash. Disappearing requires that you are able to pay for your apartment, food, clothing, and other necessities with cash only. You would never use credit cards again.

Family and friends: Your friends and family members would obviously be upset and concerned when you went missing. While it might be possible to have very limited contact with a close family member, it would have to be minimal, and it would be complicated.

Legal ramifications: Depending on where you live and what debts you have or insurance claims are made on your behalf, there could be illegalities to your disappearing.

Going alone: It would be much harder to disappear if you were unable to go alone. Disappearing with a loved one is incredibly difficult. Having additional people with you would likely lead to you eventually being caught.

What are you up against? As I've said, disappearing is a last resort and would be a viable choice only if it were the only way you could stay alive. If you were running from an abusive spouse or boyfriend, you would need to consider his or her resources. How hard would that person look for you? If you were thinking about running from the government, you'd be dealing with an entirely different ball game. The government has a virtually unlimited bank account to spend tracking you down, and running from the government would require a level of discipline that most people don't have.

Disappearing: The Three-Part Process

As you can imagine, it has never been harder to disappear. There are traces of us everywhere. Cell phones indicate exactly where we are at any time, we have credit cards, bank accounts, Social Security numbers, social media accounts, and countless other things that can lead someone right to us. According to CBS News, as many as two hundred security cameras could be watching you at any given time—surveillance cameras are found at banks, random street corners, stadiums, national monuments, and even parks. They are nearly impossible to avoid. All of this is why following each of these three steps to the letter would be crucial if you wanted to disappear without being caught.

Step 1: Misinformation

Misinformation sounds simple, but it's actually time-consuming and requires precision. Misinformation is when you purposefully manipulate the information various companies have on you. If you look in your wallet, you'll see that each credit card, membership card, and frequent flyer card holds information about you. Every time you buy something, the credit card company is listing those transactions. Every phone call you make on your cell phone or home phone is listed. You may think you've led a private and discreet life, but unless you don't have a phone and have operated on an all-cash basis, information about you is available. To begin the process of misinformation, you would start to make minor changes to every account you have. This part of the process is relatively painless, and can be completed in just a few hours. You would call every account and membership you have, and slightly change your information to throw everything off. It's not necessary to change the information drastically (you'll see why in step 2). For example, you would call your bank and change your house number, call your Visa card company and change your phone number by one digit, and so on, until you had covered every account and membership you had, including subscriptions, utilities, frequent flyer cards, and gym membership.

In addition to changing all of these, you would start giving misinformation while you're going through your daily life. For example, the next time you stopped at the dry cleaners, you would mention that you're closing your account because you're moving to Hawaii. The next time you were at the barber getting your hair cut, you'd mention that you are moving to Florida. And the next time you got on Facebook, you'd post about relocating to Alabama.

The point is to give out a bunch of false information so that no one will know where you're really going and you immediately become harder to track down.

Skip Tracers: They'll Be Looking for You
A skip tracer is a person who is hired to find someone who is missing. A skip tracer could be thought of as a combination of debt collector, bounty hunter, and private detective. If an ex-husband really wants to find you, he could use a skip tracer. If you owe someone a massive debt and have skipped town, he'd hire a skip tracer. While there are many professional skip tracers who are very good at what they do, with some perseverance and basic technical knowledge, anyone can do it. A skip tracer generally starts by collecting as much information as possible about the person he is searching for. The skip tracer will analyze and verify the

information in order to get clues about that person's whereabouts. If there is a lot of information about a person, in certain instances it may conflict, and the skip tracer will have to figure out what is accurate.

Skip tracers also use various tactics to try to get information about you out of other people. Michelle Gomez, a four-foot, eleven-inch, hundred-pound woman from Texas is considered one of the best skip tracers in the world. Gomez once needed to locate a fleet of Caterpillar wheel loaders taken by a group of Peruvians. How did she do it? Her first tactic was to find the patriarch of the family who had taken the vehicles. She contacted the patriarch's wife and told her she was carrying her husband's child. The tactic worked and she got the information she needed. Skip tracers will also use pretexting. Remember, pretexting is a form of social engineering where a person uses a false motive to obtain information about someone. A skip tracer might call the bank pretending to be you. They might say, "Hey, I didn't get my bank statement this month, can you confirm you sent it to this address?" The bank employee may very well say "No. We sent it to 123 Sycamore Street." And now the skip tracer has your home address. You want to be especially careful about pretexts conducted by women. Society is conditioned to feel more comfortable divulging information to women. If a man calls up and asks for a phone number, a person might be scared off, and won't give it. If it's a woman, it can be a different story. I was once in a situation in which I needed to get some information from a reporter. I knew it wouldn't be easy for me, so I asked an attractive female friend to help out. Not only did she get the information I needed, she was asked out on a date (the guy was married; she said no). This just shows how conditioned we are as a society to let our guards down for women.

Step 2: Disinformation

Disinformation is key if you want to keep the skip tracers off your back. The purpose of disinformation is to manipulate people. You want them wondering what's true. What information can be trusted? If you wanted to keep a skip tracer really busy, you could create different trails of false information. They'd have to investigate each trail, ideally finding that none of them lead back to you. For the purposes of disappearing, your goal would be to spread false information about yourself and the place where you are moving.

Investigate Your New City

If you currently live in Milwaukee, but wanted to disappear, you could give off the impression that you're moving to Arizona. How would you do this? By flying out to Arizona just like you would if you were really relocating. You'd look at apartments and houses. You'd go through the motions of signing a lease. You would want your skip tracer to report back to your ex-husband or whoever that your "credit was checked by ABC Realty Company in Arizona." You could rent a post office box, have packages or mail sent, or even rent a place to live (obviously that would require serious financial resources). The bottom line is you would need to leave a trail in your new city, providing evidence that you were really moving there, and you would need to make it as convincing as possible. As you can see, disinformation takes a lot of work because you'd have to go to that city and do everything that a person who was truly going to live in that city would do.

Step 3: Reformation

You might have guessed right away that if you're fleeing from your ex-husband in Milwaukee, you're not really moving to Arizona. After setting up your PO box and having your credit checked by rental agencies in Arizona, you would actually be moving to a totally different city. For this case, let's say you made it look like you were moving to Phoenix, but Philadelphia is the city you really plan to move to. How would you get there? You wouldn't fly or travel in any way that could be traced. You would take buses and trains, and meander your way to Philadelphia. You might stop in Chicago, and then Pittsburgh, or even go out of your way and get to New York City before heading west to Philadelphia.

Money

Whitey Bulger, the infamous crime boss who spent sixteen years in hiding, had $822,198 in cash hidden in the walls of the apartment he shared in Santa Monica, California, with Catherine Greig. The seemingly innocent retirees paid for the monthly rent at the Princess Eugenia apartments in cash. The landlord never suspected a thing. When disappearing, it's best to operate on an all-cash basis, for obvious reasons. Clearly this is difficult to do, but if you were staying off the grid you'd have to find a way to live without credit cards, ID, and a Social Security number. Prepaid credit cards used to be a great option, but now the U.S. government tracks everything, so cash is the only way you wouldn't leave any type of trail. If you needed extra money, you'd have to get an under-the-table job, such as working in a mom and pop restaurant or maybe in construction.

Just Like the President, You'll Never Drive Again

When Ellen DeGeneres asked former President Bill Clinton what he used to do every day in normal life that he missed the most, he immediately answered, "Drive." President Obama referred to driving a Chevrolet Volt about ten feet in the GM plant as a "joyride." Both presidents have been known to enjoy driving golf carts. Driving is a freedom most of us take for granted. We drive every day without thinking about what it would be like if we couldn't do it anymore. If you were planning to disappear, you would have to say good-bye to driving, and you'd have to opt for an area where you could get what you need by walking or public transportation. It's just too dangerous to risk getting pulled over. If you're pulled over, you've basically been discovered.

After five years in hiding, it was getting pulled over for drunk driving that got a wanted criminal caught. Fingerprints showed that the guy who got pulled over by the Vegas police was actually a man who was wanted for perpetrating a $100 million pyramid scheme. Driving is one of the surest ways to get caught. It's just too easy to get pulled over for a traffic violation or even have a minor accident.

Habits Need to Be Broken

Our habits give away more clues about us than we'd think. For example, it's very easy to discover that I'm a gun enthusiast. If I ever had to disappear, I know that I would not be able to visit shooting ranges or go to a local gun store, because that is the first place that people would look for me. In the search for Whitey Bulger, authorities tried to use the couple's known love of animals as a clue, and questioned area veterinarians. Anyone who knows you is going to be familiar with your passions—and you'd have to make a point of giving up some of the activities you love the most in order to stay missing. If your ex-boyfriend knows you hit the yoga studio nearly every day, he's going to hope to find you in one. This can be one of the biggest challenges in reformation—truly turning yourself into a new person. That's why it's essential you remember that every time you engage in an activity from your previous life, you are leaving clues for whoever is looking for you.

Communication: Tricky, but Not Impossible

The Prepaid Cell Phone

These days it's incredibly easy to track someone down who has a regular cell phone. Obviously if you were disappearing, you would have ditched your smartphone. The good news is that there is a safe and inexpensive way you could have minimal contact with family members; however, this depends on the level of the threat against you. If you were running from an ex who has lots of resources, I have to say, it's best to never touch a cell phone or speak to your family again. If your threat was not that high, then you could use a prepaid cell phone. The prepaid cell phone is an incredibly handy device, and they are easy to find. All you would need to do is buy a prepaid cell phone (using cash), along with a card full of minutes. These are available at your typical big box stores. You'd just take it up to the counter and have it activated. You would also want them to install the minutes for you. But remember, when the store clerk asks you if you want to associate an email address or phone number with the phone, *the answer would be no*. Once your phone was activated, you could use it to safely call your family. To be extra safe, I'd replace the phone from time to time—discarding the old ones.

The Break Phone

If you were running from the mafia, Mexican drug cartels, or you're seriously concerned your ex-husband was going to harm you, then you would never touch a cell phone again. But if you insisted on staying in touch with someone and the threat was incredibly high, you would want to take it up a step higher with cell phones. A break phone enables you to safely place a phone call by using a third phone. It's a process that involves three prepaid phones. Here's how you would do it:

1. Go to a store and buy one prepaid cell phone (using cash) and have them activate it for you.
2. Go to another store and buy a second prepaid phone.
3. And go to a third store and buy a third prepaid phone, so you now have a total of three phones.
4. Take the first prepaid phone (*phone one*) and give it to the friend or family member that you've insisted on staying in contact with. Make sure you write down the phone number so you know the number to reach them at.
5. Take the second prepaid phone (*phone two*) and set up call forwarding on it so that it automatically forwards to phone one. In other words, if anyone calls the second phone it immediately forwards to the first phone you've given to your family member. Once call forwarding is set up on phone two, you destroy phone two. Smash it in a thousand pieces and throw it in a river.
6. Phone three is the phone you use to call phone two, which automatically forwards on to phone one. I know this can be a little confusing, but you've essentially put a middleman between you so that no one can track you

(not even the National Security Agency). Just remember, only you can call your loved one; he or she cannot call you. The phones would need to be replaced frequently, at least once a month.

The break phone is high-level serious stuff, and I certainly hope you would never need to use it.

Computers and Social Media

Hopefully I don't need to tell you that social media is off limits. Skip Tracer Michelle Gomez told *Wired* magazine that the people she chases understand that to avoid getting caught, you have to work hard to limit your digital trail. This means staying off of computers and using Facebook only to plant false information at the very beginning before you relocate.

The Disappearing Email

If you were disappearing, you would need to stay off computers. But if the threat level isn't very high, there is a way to send an email with an address that disappears. Guerrilla Mail gives you a disposable email address. You don't even have to register on the site. The email address that is generated for you disappears within an hour after you've sent the message.

Live the Disguise: How to Become Invisible

In April 2003, when Scott Peterson was arrested by the San Diego police in La Jolla, California, his appearance had changed. Peterson had bleached his hair and goatee. Rather than admit he was trying to disguise himself, Petersen claimed his hair was bleached by chlorine in a friend's swimming pool. (Even more suspicious were the items Peterson had on him at the time of his arrest. Peterson had $1,000 in cash, four cell phones, credit cards that belonged to members of his family, camping equipment and survival gear, and his brother's driver's license.) Peterson's disguise was terrible because not only was he still recognizable but the bleached blond hair made him stand out even more than his regular hair color had. The purpose of a disguise is to make you look as boring and bland as possible so you don't stand out from the crowd.

New Hair Color Is Not Enough

A good disguise must do more than make you unrecognizable. A disguise must be comprehensive, so that everything you carry—from what's in your wallet to what's in your coat pockets—supports your new persona. The most effective disguises also render you *unnoticeable*. Whitey Bulger and Catherine Greig were known as just a "very nice old couple." Residents of their apartment complex said the couple took walks on the beach or in the park, and took care of stray cats. Nothing unusual about that. That's so typical they're basically invisible. This is what you would hope to achieve when taking on a new persona after disappearing. You'd want to think about what kinds of jobs and personalities blend into the scenery—neighborhood housewife who gardens, garbage collector, waiter at a local restaurant. You would want to put yourself in the position of going unnoticed and not thought about at all.

Studio Six Productions: You're a Big-Time Hollywood Producer

Perhaps the most famous disguises of all time were created by ex–CIA officer Tony Mendez (who was later played by Ben Affleck in the movie *Argo*). Mendez had spent fourteen years in the CIA's Office of Technical Services when he found himself tasked with getting six Americans out of the Canadian Embassy during the Iran Hostage Crisis. Mendez had a specialty of using "identity transformation" to get people out of really difficult situations. Knowing whatever tactic he took to get the Americans out would have to slip under the radar, Mendez decided he'd have to create a situation that enabled the Americans to take on false identities, walk through the airport and simply get on a plane. After pondering a few scenarios, such as pretending the Americans were teachers, or nutritionists inspecting crops—it became clear that the only scenario that might work was actually pretty crazy. Mendez worked with some contacts in Hollywood to establish Studio Six Productions. At the time, no one who wasn't directly involved knew that the "Six" referred to the six Americans whose lives Mendez was trying to save. Mendez planned to pretend the six Americans were part of a location-scouting party checking out Iran as a potential set.

The operation had to look legit, and every detail was considered. A script was acquired that featured a setting that potentially resembled Iran. Business cards were created, former movie credits were made for each of the scouting party. The business office of the studio (which they rented in Hollywood) had multiple phone lines, including one with an unpublished number strictly for CIA purposes. Ads were taken out in *Variety*. Studio Six Productions started receiving scripts and headshots—and questions about when the movie *Argo* would be shot. Bob Sidell, one of the producers helping Mendez out, even took meetings to hear pitches from producers about other movies Studio Six Production should consider making.

Once Mendez made it into Iran, he pitched the idea to the Americans, and handed out their new Canadian identities. Mendez worked with the Canadian government to get real passports, and health cards were given out. Driver's licenses and fake receipts for random purchases were distributed. Even Canadian maple leaf pins were on hand. The Americans learned the storyline and rehearsed their roles. In the car on their way to the airport, Cora Lijek, the American Foreign Service worker who was now "Teresa Harris the writer," double-checked her pockets for anything that might have her real name. After a harrowing wait at the airport, the Americans made it onto the plane and ended up toasting each other with Bloody Marys. The third, unpublished phone line back at Studio Six Productions finally rang, alerting the production studio that the Americans had made it out.

While the story of *Argo* is undeniably dramatic, there are some basic disguise concepts highlighted here that can make the difference between escaping unnoticed and being discovered.

Know Who You're Trying to Be

If your goal is to disappear, your disguise would need to go beyond hair color and clothes—you'd have to change who you are. When coming up with a new persona, you would want to think of options that while different from what you currently do, are in fact doable. It might be possible to pull yourself off as a chef—but think twice before announcing you're a brain surgeon. If you're a lawyer, you would want to stick with an identity that's close to that. You wouldn't want to try to pull yourself off as a plumber, especially if you know nothing about what being a plumber entails, or what a plumber carries around with him on a daily basis. Mendez flew to Hollywood and met with select people he had known from the industry and got information before setting up a fake production company. He made sure the six Americans understood what their various jobs in the production company entailed. You would need to do some homework, too.

Find the Baseline

Hopefully by now you're learning how important it would be to blend in to your surroundings. Whatever you'd be wearing to complete your disguise would need to make sense as part of the environment you're living in. A cowboy hat might go unnoticed in Dallas, Texas, but it would to stick out like crazy in Chicago. Take a look around and note what regular people are wearing. Make sure your choices fall in line and that you don't stand out. I do a fun exercise during my Spy Escape and Evasion classes in Las Vegas. We'll check out what people are wearing at high-end hotels such as the Wynn, and then at the less expensive hotels such as the Riviera. It might be normal to see jeans, sneakers, and a sweatshirt at the buffet at the Riviera. That same outfit is not going to fly at an A-list party in a nightclub at the Wynn. Check out the details as well. What kinds of handbags are women carrying? What kinds of coats do people wear? Fleece? Raincoats? Trench coats? And don't forget to pay attention to shoes. It's easy to forget that your shoes are a key part of your disguise. If no one wears heels where you're living, don't be the one person who wears heels to the grocery store.

Hide Your Most Recognizable Features

If you were trying to disappear, you might finally regret that tattoo you got in college. Any distinguishing characteristics would need to be disguised. You might need to cover a tattoo or even have your teeth fixed. If you're bald, you'd need a convincing wig. If you have a mole, you would need to get it removed. If everyone associates you with your funky glasses, you'd need to give them up and consider contact lenses. We all have physical characteristics that are associated strongly with our appearances. Think carefully about any features you have that stand out, and consider options for playing them down.

Change Your Features

Hair

Countless movies show people changing their appearances by cutting their hair. Julia Roberts cut off her auburn locks when fleeing her violent husband in *Sleeping with the Enemy*. In the movie based on the hit book *Gone Girl*, Amy Dunne dyes her hair darker and cuts it to chin length. It seems like it could be trivial, but changing your hair is one of the easiest and quickest changes you can make to your appearance. Change your cut, dye it, and try out wigs and hair extensions. While changing hairstyles may seem more challenging for men, you can alter your appearance by changing the shape of your facial hair or even better, completely shaving it off.

Size and Posture

You'd be amazed how your size, height, and posture play a key role in your appearance. Alter your posture, make a point of slouching or carry yourself differently from how you normally do. Over time, losing or gaining weight can also help make a person less recognizable.

Abandon Your Regular Style—Permanently

If everyone in town can recognize you because you're always wearing a Green Bay Packers sweatshirt and baseball cap, you would need to stop showing your team spirit. If you've worn sneakers, T-shirt, and jeans every day for the past twenty years, switching to khakis and a polo shirt would be a start in throwing people off (but only if it fits into the baseline of your new community). On the flip side, if you're a suit guy, you could embrace shorts and a baggy shirt. It's possible to disguise yourself further by changing the fit of your clothes. If you usually favor looser styles, people may have no idea that underneath those baggy clothes you're actually tall and lean.

Building a Disguise Kit

If you wanted to disappear, you would need to gather items to help conceal your identity. The following could help you create a disguise for your new persona:

- Wigs
- Fake mustaches, goatees, and moles
- Temporary tattoos
- Sunglasses

Disguise on the Run

If you needed to go on the run at a moment's notice, you could disguise yourself and avoid being recognized by security cameras quite easily. It can take as little as a hat, a pair of glasses, and some clothes you wouldn't normally wear to escape notice.

- Hats and baseball caps
- Nonprescription glasses
- Fake eyelashes
- Clip-on earrings
- Fake piercings
- Clothing that fits whoever you were trying to be—hippie, conservative businessman, sports fanatic (subtle is best)
- Contacts
- Makeup
- Hair extensions
- Wedding ring (if you wanted to appear unmarried, you would take your ring off in advance, to allow time for the dent on your finger to go away)
- Jewelry and watches

The Art of Pocket Litter

Cora Lijek, one of the women who escaped Iran disguised as a screenwriter, was right to check her pockets for evidence that would give her true identity away. The contents of pockets, wallets, and purses are an important part of pulling off a disguise. If you were to look in your pockets, wallet, purse, or at the stuff in your car, there are probably a few things that give away quite a bit of information about you. An empty Starbucks cup tells me you drink coffee, a receipt from a bookstore suggests you like to read, and the crushed Goldfish crackers on the floor of your car are a definite sign of having kids. When planning a disguise, you would need to think about the kinds of items the person you've transformed into would be carrying. If I were trying to pass myself off as a movie producer, I'd probably have a cell phone, business cards, and receipts from fancy restaurants. If I were a construction worker I might have a screwdriver, utility knife blade, and nails. Disguises need to be thorough, and carrying the appropriate materials with you at all times is important.

Identification

One of the biggest challenges to disappearing off the face of the earth is dealing with identification. As I've said, truly disappearing means giving up activities that require a government-issued ID. You won't be getting on planes or driving anymore. Again, this is something that needs to be seriously considered before taking steps to disappear. Here's some additional information about IDs I think everyone should know.

Never Get a "Government-Issued" Fake ID

If you were trying to disappear, it might be tempting to find someone who will forge a passport or driver's license for you. Know that

HOW TO DISAPPEAR WITHOUT A TRACE   197

if you did this, you'd get caught. It's extremely difficult to get a fake government-issued ID. Holograms and magnetic strips have made them nearly impossible to reproduce. Should you be tempted to get one online, know it's a scam. If you send away $500 to get a fake California driver's license, I guarantee you'll never see that money again, and that ID isn't coming. It's also illegal.

Company IDs

I am sometimes hired to do a building penetration. If you've ever seen the movie *Sneakers* then you know what this is. It's basically my job to see how easy it is to get into a place I'm not really supposed to be. Whenever I do this, I see firsthand how conditioned people are to accept a company ID. One time I was trying to get into a convention. All I did was make a cheap and easy ID with a lanyard. I just walked up to the security guy and said, "Hey, looks like it's going to be a long day." He basically replied "Yeah," saw my "company ID," and let me right in. The ID I made worked, but I also acted like I was *supposed to be there*. I approached the guy and started a conversation. I wasn't skulking around, acting nervous and like I was up to no good.

You certainly don't want to be doing anything illegal, but if your inner spy wanted to have some fun by making a company ID, all you would need are a few cheap items and a little bit of time. I'd also like to point out that you should certainly never accept a stranger's company ID without verifying who she is and why she's there. If FedEx arrives with a package or someone from a util-

> *Never accept a stranger's company ID without verifying who she is and why she's there.*

ity company shows up at your door, look up the number and call
to confirm (it's important that you get the number yourself).

Your Inner Clark Kent/Superman

As I've said, I hope and expect that you'll never need to disappear.
On the off chance you need to pull off a disguise, you can draw
inspiration from an unlikely source—Navey Baker, a tomboyish
Mormon teenage girl from Texas. Baker describes herself as shy
and quiet. She even feels uncomfortable ordering a burrito at
Taco Bell. But Baker also compares herself to Superman, basically
acquiring powers when she puts on her "disguise," which is a
giant tiger costume. Baker is the beloved school mascot of the
Gilbert High School Tigers football team. NPR's *This American
Life* profiled Baker and her ability to completely transform her
personality by putting on a disguise. Baker said that by putting
on a tiger costume, she becomes someone who "doesn't care." In
her disguise, the shy teenager has been described as having "serious swagger." When Baker is wearing her disguise, she can do
cartwheels—something she is completely incapable of doing in
her normal state. While you might not expect a self-proclaimed
awkward teenager to be a role model for those who want to
conceal their identity, her ability to transform her personality
exemplifies disguise wearing at its best.

11

THE ART OF SURVIVAL DRIVING

About five years ago, I was driving through Baltimore. It was after a massive snowstorm, and there weren't any other cars on the road. I was driving down a narrow city street, each side lined with row houses. Suddenly a guy ran right up to my car, and tried to open the door. He couldn't get it open because I always make a point of locking my doors. I immediately accelerated and brought my eyes back to the road in front of me. A woman was standing right in front of my car, trying to block me in. Thanks to the training I've had, I was able to swerve around her and get away. When I looked in my rearview mirror as I sped off, about ten people had rushed out into the street, intent on chasing down my car. While I was fortunate enough to get away, things don't end so well for everyone.

At about 9 p.m. on a Sunday a few weeks before Christmas, thirty-year-old Dustin Friedland and his wife, Jamie, were headed back to their Range Rover after shopping at an upscale New Jersey mall. Mr. Friedland closed the passenger side door for his wife when he was suddenly jumped by four men. There was a confrontation and Mr. Friedland was shot in the head (he was later pronounced dead at a local hospital). His wife was forced out of the car by one of the men, and they fled the scene. The men who stole the vehicle ended up abandoning it in nearby Newark. It turns out that the four men involved in the carjacking had serious criminal histories and had spent time in prison for multiple burglaries and drug counts.

One of Tennessee's most grisly crimes began with a carjacking. Christopher Newsom and Channon Christian had been dating just a couple of months when they decided to go out for dinner. When neither of them returned home, their families called the police. Police soon found out that a railroad worker had found Newsom's body near some tracks outside of Knoxville. Eventually Christian's body was discovered as well. When the situation was pieced together by authorities, they were able to determine that the couple had been carjacked in an apartment building parking lot. While thankfully most carjacking victims do not suffer anywhere near as terrible a fate as the young couple did, carjacking is a serious crime that you must be prepared to combat.

A Serious Threat

Carjacking, basically a serious and possibly life-threatening form of car theft, is currently the fastest growing crime in America. Cars have become much more complicated to break into, and as a result, it's simply easier for a criminal to steal a car directly from an individual by using force. I want you to know a few statistics about carjacking:

- 77% of carjackings involve a weapon, most often a gun.
- 87% of carjackings are committed by men.
- 54% of carjackings are committed by two or more people.
- A carjacker is most likely going to be a male under the age of twenty-nine.
- Most carjackings occur during the evening or late at night.
- Most carjackings take place in urban areas, followed by suburban, then rural areas.
- 63% of carjackings occur within five miles of the victim's home.
- Carjackings are most likely to take place on a Sunday night.

And while I can tell you firsthand that being the victim of an attempted carjacking is a scary ordeal, there are many simple things you can do to stay safe in your car.

Survival Driving Basics

Before we get into some of the admittedly more exciting aspects of survival driving, you need to be aware of the incredibly simple tactics that can save your life. I know what I'm about to tell you will sound like simple common sense, but you'd be surprised by how many people don't do these things. Everything I'm about to talk about should become second nature, like putting on your seat belt.

Lock Your Doors

In Houston, a woman was carjacked while stopped at a red light. The assistant police chief told the local news that the criminal "opened the door and got in." Once he was in the vehicle, the armed criminal ordered the woman to drive to an abandoned restaurant, where he told her to get out. The vehicle was later tracked down via the GPS on her OnStar system. If you don't already, you need to get in the habit of immediately locking your doors once you get in the car.

Windows Up

A Seattle area man probably regrets keeping the windows down while he sat in his parked car, waiting for his wife. He was playing on his iPad, but soon decided to put his iPad between the seats, close his eyes and meditate.

Moments later, he felt something touch his leg. A teenaged boy had reached his hand in through a side window and stolen his iPad.

While it's clearly not a good idea to sit back in your car with your eyes closed with the windows down, it's absolutely critical not to open your window for anyone. It was around 11 p.m. when "Danny" (the twenty-six-year-old entrepreneur did not wish to use his real name) pulled his car over to the side of the road to answer a text. A car swerved behind his, slamming on the brakes. A man got out of the car and knocked on his window, and unfortunately, Danny decided to open it to see what the man wanted. At that point, the man reached into the car and unlocked it. He entered the car, and was carrying a silver handgun. This wasn't just a carjacking—it was a carjacking by a high-profile criminal, who was currently being hunted by authorities. Danny was ordered to drive, and when the moment was right, he acted quickly. They were stopped at a gas station that had a sign reading "cash only." While the younger brother went inside to pay, Danny simply unbuckled his seat belt, opened the door and sprinted off. He was able to make it to a gas station across the street, where he hid in a supply room and asked the clerk to call 911.

While Danny's story is unusual, it's all too easy to be a target when you're stopped at a light or parked with your windows open. Driving with your window open or opening it to speak with a stranger makes you immediately vulnerable to robbery or carjacking. Resist the temptation to drive with your windows down. It's just not worth it.

Turn Your Car Off

Life is busy, and it's really easy to think it will be OK to pop into a store to run a quick errand or chat with a friend without turning your car off. There's a father in Minneapolis who learned the hard way how bad an idea this is. A man was at a gas station when he saw an acquaintance. He got out of his car to talk to the person, leaving his car unlocked, with his two-year-old son in the backseat. All of a sudden, a person got into his car and sped away. Thankfully, the police found the car a short time later, with the sleeping child safely inside. Residents of Colorado Springs have seen a rash of running vehicles stolen while they're being warmed up, with their owners remaining in their homes. In Baltimore, law-enforcement officials were surprised to discover that half of all cars stolen in

Baltimore had their keys left in the ignition. The *Baltimore Sun* points out that this problem isn't unique to Baltimore. The National Highway Traffic Safety Administration and U.S. Department of Transportation estimate that 40 to 50 percent of vehicle theft is the result of driver error. This means either leaving the keys in the ignition or leaving doors un-

40 to 50 percent of vehicle theft is the result of driver error.

locked with the keys on the seat. As we discussed in Chapter 1, most crimes are crimes of opportunity. Don't make it easier for potential thieves to steal your vehicle by leaving your door open and the keys inside. Always take the extra few seconds to turn your car off, even if you're in your own driveway. The alternative—running quickly into your house to get your wallet, and coming out to find your car stolen—isn't worth the risk.

As Always, Practice Situational Awareness

It's easy to think you're secure in your car because it's your own personal space. The bottom line is that when you're in your car, you need to remain in Condition Yellow, just as you would if you were walking down the street. Susan Biggs, a Florida-based nurse, was reading in the parking lot of a hospital before her shift started. While she was reading, two men approached her open window. They had a gun, and told her to get out of the car. The suspects fled the scene with her car. They were caught after a long chase. It's unfortunate that you can't behave in your car as you would in your home, but that is the world we live in today.

When You're Most Vulnerable

Make a point of being extra vigilant when you are stopped at a light or a stop sign. Obviously, if your car isn't moving, you're an easy target. When you're pushing 75 miles per hour down the highway you're not an easy target and don't have to worry about someone carjacking you. If someone approaches your car, do not roll down the window or attempt to talk to them. Keep an eye on his hands and what he is doing. If you see him reach for a knife or a gun or if your gut instinct tells you something isn't right, then drive somewhere—whether it's to the left or right or backward or forward. Remember, *movement saves lives*, so get yourself out of the danger zone.

You Don't Have to Be in Your Car

Remember, carjackings can take place inside or outside of your vehicle. Dustin Friedland wasn't in his car when the deadly carjacking took place. He was approaching his vehicle after exiting a shopping mall. When you're walking to your car, be aware of places where someone may be hiding, park in well-lit areas, and always have your keys ready.

Can You See the Tires?

The next time you're stopped at a light, take a moment to observe the car in front of you. How close are you actually stopped to that car? Can you see the tires? Teach yourself to stop at a point that enables you to see the tires of the vehicle in front of you. This is an important safety precaution that can save your life. Every time you

Be sure to take control of the space in front of you.

are stopped or stuck in traffic, be sure to stop your vehicle before you are too close to see the tires. Leaving this amount of space enables you to get around that vehicle should you need to get away in an emergency. You can't do anything to control the space behind your car, so be sure to take control of the space in front of you.

Your Gas Tank

You've all heard that you should always have at least a half tank of gas. I realize that isn't always easy to do and that most people will never do it. However, do not let your car get below a quarter of a tank—and never let it get so low that the gas light goes on. If something happens, and you're in an evasive driving situation, a quarter of a tank can get you about seventy miles. That's far enough to get you out of a potentially dangerous situation.

Tires = Control

I cannot stress enough how important it is to have quality, properly maintained tires on your vehicle. Four tires are all that's between you, your loved ones, and the road. If you are ever in an evasive driving situation, you're going to need as much control as you can get, and this is going to come from your tires. And when was the last time you checked the air pressure on your tires? It turns out that most of us are driving with underinflated tires. Here's a rule of thumb to follow: *Keep your tires 10 percent under the recommended pounds per square inch (psi) given on the tire wall.* In other words, if you go out to your car today and it says forty-four psi on the tire wall, then you would inflate your tires to forty. (I'm not concerned with what the manufacturer of the car says, because they don't know which tires you may end up putting on the vehicle.) Not only will you have better control, but you'll get better gas mileage. Once you get your tires at the optimum pressure, make a point of checking your tire pressure from time to time. And don't forget to check your spare tire.

The Right Adjustments

One of the first things I do when I teach my Escape & Evasion Driving Experience (SpyDriving.com), is show people how to know if their seat is in the optimum position for driving. Many people are actually sitting too far away from the steering wheel. There's a simple thing you can do to see where your seat should be. The next time you get into your car, put your arm straight out toward the steering wheel and rest your arm on top of the steering wheel. You want the bottom of your wrist to rest on top of the steering wheel. If your fingers are touching the wheel then you are too far back and you need to move your seat forward. If the steering wheel is touching your forearm then move it back until your wrist is what's resting on the steering wheel with your arm fully extended.

Hand Position

People who have taken my class know what a difference proper hand positioning makes. We do a series of drills evading roadblocks and ramming vehicles. People discover right away that if your hands aren't positioned at *nine and three o'clock*, you can't get

One Hollywood Cliché That's True: The Panel Van

We've all seen a movie where someone gets grabbed, and shoved into a van. This is one of the few clichés I can tell you is true. A woman who took my class had a horrifying near encounter with a panel van. It was a bright afternoon, in a nice part of LA. She was walking down the street when she noticed a white panel van driving next to her. She was immediately uncomfortable. All of a sudden a guy grabbed her wrist. Luckily she knew what to do and fought him off while she screamed like crazy. The guy jumped into the van and drove off. Numerous similar examples exist, both in the United States and abroad. There's a reason for this. It's a lot easier to shove someone, particularly someone large, into a van than trying to get him or her into a regular car. So even though it's become a cliché, keep your distance.

enough control over the car to properly execute maneuvers. Should you ever end up in an evasive driving situation, it's critical your hands are in this position. Having your hands at nine and three o'clock automatically forces you to keep your elbows bent, which enables you to get the most mobility out of your car. If your hands are in these positions, and there's a guy standing in front of your car trying to block you, you're easily going to be able to maneuver your car around him.

Your Side Mirrors

Most Americans use their side mirrors to see the back of their cars. The next time you get in your car, look in your side mirrors. If you can see any part of the back of your car, you need to push them out. This will give you more peripheral vision when you're driving, and you'll be able to see what's in your blind spot better.

Carjacking: How It Can Happen

In some cases, carjackers simply approach the car, show their weapons, and demand you get out. Other times, carjackers will use trickier methods to manipulate you into a position where your car can be stolen. By being aware of the various tactics used by carjackers, you'll know when a situation might not be quite what it seems.

The Bump and Rob

It's natural to want to be diligent and make sure no damage was done to your car in a fender bender. If you find yourself in a situation where the person behind you bumps into your car, you might want to think twice about inspecting the damage. In Delray Beach, Florida, a man got cash from a bank and was then rear-ended. When the man got out to inspect the damage, two men got out of the car, pulled out a handgun and bound the victim's wrists and demanded money. When the man claimed he had no money, one of the robbers pulled cash out of the man's shirt. The other robber tried to get into the man's car, but the doors were locked. A similar situation in Atlanta, Georgia, ended tragically. Fifty-three-year-old

Janice Pitts was driving to work with her daughter and four-year-old grandson when she was hit several times by Dewey Green at a light. When she got out to examine her car, Green accelerated his car, pinning the grandmother between the two vehicles. Green then backed his truck up, gunned his car, and drove over Pitts, killing her. Green had a history of reckless driving, sealed drug arrests, and a record of criminal mischief as a minor.

The Good Samaritan, the Carjacking Version

We've already talked about how being a Good Samaritan can get you into trouble. The same thing goes for potential carjackers. Four teenage girls in Orlando thought faking car trouble would be a great way to get money for gas and going out for a night on the town. The girls drove around with their hazard lights on, and when they noticed a young man walking along the street, they pulled into a parking lot and asked for help with their overheating car. Twenty-one-year-old Cameron Castro popped the hood, and one of the girls covered her face with her shirt and asked for "everything he had." Castro handed over $50, only to get struck twice by the front bumper of the car. In Greenville, Tennessee, three suspects also faked road trouble to lure Good Samaritans. Apparently a male and female suspect sat on the side of the highway with the hood of their car up. The woman was holding what appeared to be a baby and was gesturing for help. When someone stopped to help, a man got out of the SUV, and the two men approached the victims with guns while demanding money.

It's completely understandable to want to help victims of a car accident, but it's also possible that the accident could be rigged. The bottom line is, if you see someone who looks like he needs help, use your cell phone to call the police, but if you decide to get out and help, be extremely cautious.

The Trap

The trap is basically a way of robbing you in your own driveway. Leamon R. Hunt, a U.S. diplomat, was assassinated in Rome in 1984 in a variation of the trap. One night, Hunt arrived at his home, where he had to wait for a gate to open before driving onto his property. While he was waiting, three gunmen emerged from a car parked across the street and opened fire. Hunt was ultimately killed when a gunman jumped onto the trunk of his limousine and fired a shot that went through a gap in the bulletproof glass of his vehicle.

The Ruse

We all want to be safe drivers, so if another driver is flashing his lights at us, or gesturing at us to pull over, we may do so out of concern for our safety. However, carjackers have been known to prey on these fears to put people in a vulnerable position. If someone is waving frantically for you to pull over and your car isn't on fire, and nothing appears to be wrong, just call the police and keep going.

How to Avoid Being Carjacked

While there are some basic tactics you can take to stay safer while driving, keep in mind that carjackers can get creative, and you must remain alert and aware. In England, carjackers started leaving brochures on the back windows of cars. Drivers didn't really notice the papers until they begin driving, and looked out their rear window. When the driver pulls over to remove the annoying piece of paper, carjackers are hopping into the front seat and pulling off. So, remember to practice situational awareness at all times, and practice the following tactics:

- Always keep your windows up and doors locked.
- Practice avoidance. Do not drive in high-crime areas or isolated areas and try to avoid driving late at night.
- Be especially vigilant when stopped at red lights or in traffic jams. As always, do not talk on your phone, send messages, or play games on your smartphone.
- Any minor damage your vehicle may incur due to a minor traffic accident is not worth risking your life. Don't be concerned about minor damage in a fender bender. It's perfectly fine to simply put on your flashers and call the police, and stay inside your car until an officer arrives on the scene.
- Don't risk your own safety by being a Good Samaritan on the side of the road or on a major highway, regardless of the situation. If you want to help, simply call 911 and report that there are individuals on the side of the road who require assistance.
- If someone approaches your window and wants to talk to you, talk through the window, but do not open it. The window provides a psychological barrier as well as a physical one. It will feel weird, but most likely the criminal will see that you aren't a good target, and will leave.

- Keep a cell phone in your car should you need to call for help.
- Listen to your gut, as I urge you to do in any situation. In my line of work, I've come across many people who have been carjacked. All of these people have told me "something just didn't feel right." Follow your instincts.
- You already know that it's crucial to make sure no one is following you in your vehicle. Get in the habit of checking your rearview mirror before you take that final turn to your home. If you ever suspect someone is following you, keep moving and call the police.
- Resist the urge to organize belongings when you get in your car. Try not to spend time putting items in your purse. Fiddling with your GPS system or making calls puts you in a vulnerable position. Look up frequently if you must do things in your car before driving off.
- Think like a criminal. Do you look like a good target? Are you talking on your cell phone as you leave the mall? Are you wearing lots of expensive jewelry? It should be noted that carjackers are interested in women, both young and old—who are alone. They aren't interested in groups of people, because they're much harder to handle. And, it might make some of you feel better to know that carjackers are unlikely to target mothers who are with their children. Mothers will fight like crazy, so they are generally avoided.

How to Handle a Carjacking

While I certainly hope you will never be the victim of a carjacking, I'm going to tell you exactly what to do should the unthinkable happen. You're stopped at a red light when an armed criminal approaches you and demands your car. What should you do? I'm going to remind you once again that *movement saves lives*. Whatever you do, make sure freezing is not your response.

If You're with a Child

Do not ask permission to get your child. Simply tell the carjackers your child is in the car and you are getting him. Go to your child, remove him from the seat belt and exit the car.

If a Carjacker Tries to Take You

It is important that you know that you are in danger of losing your life if you get into a car with a criminal. Your chances of being raped or killed go up substantially if you get in a car with a criminal. Do not believe movies you see in Hollywood where people get in cars with criminals, and talk the criminal into letting them go. If you are being forced into a car, fight in any way you can to avoid this happening. Use your gun, knife, tactical pen, or whatever you have and do whatever you need to in order to make sure you don't end up riding away with the carjacker.

Your Car Goes Where Your Eyes Go

Ever seen a drunk driver on the news who managed to hit the one tree in a big field? Or the one light post in a big parking lot? This is because your car goes where your eyes go, and this is important to know when doing evasive driving maneuvers. For example, should you ever find yourself having to do evasive maneuvers in a foreign country where roads are narrower, make sure you keep your eyes on the place in the road where you need to turn, and you'll have a much easier time maneuvering your car in the correct places.

Your Inner Spy: Evasive Driving Maneuvers

When most people think of spy movies, they think of car chases— cars being chased by helicopters, cars flying off bridges, spies shooting at bad guys out of windows while flying through busy cities. One of my favorite classes to teach is the Escape & Evasion Driving Experience, where everyday Americans learn how to do a 180-reverse turn, avoid an ambush, ram a vehicle, and much, much more. Here are a few of the tips that I share with my students that may save your life one day:

The Reverse 180, or the *Rockford Files* Reverse

Maybe you remember the crazy maneuvers Jim Rockford did in his gold Pontiac Firebird. Somehow that guy was always getting himself in situations where the reverse 180 was the only option. So what do you do if you need to drive backward in order to go forward?

1. Put your *left* hand in the *nine o'clock position*.
2. Drive backward toward the spot where you need to turn around. To ensure your car ends up in the reverse position, you need to be going at least 20 miles per hour and you'll want to go between 20 and 30 miles per hour.
3. When you hit the area in the road where you want to turn around, whip your left hand immediately to the *three o'clock position* while simultaneously *taking your foot off of the gas*. You should not have a foot on the gas pedal or the brake at this point.
4. Your front end will spin around and you should now be facing in the opposite direction. *Shift the car into drive*, and continue driving until you are safe. (If you want to see a video of ABC's *Shark Tank* star Daymond John doing this 180-reverse turn, visit SpyDriving.com.)

The Killzone Drill

This is a technique I teach to people who are in the executive protection business. Imagine a scenario where you're in a convoy and one of the cars gets disabled during an attack. Using a car that is still running, you need to push the disabled car out of the area of attack.

1. You're going to steer in unison with the person who remains in the disabled car. Their car must be in neutral.
2. Do not mash down on the gas pedal. You want to drive slowly in reverse until you make contact with the disabled car.
3. Once you've made contact, continue driving in reverse, pushing the other car to safety.

How to Ram a Car

Imagine a scenario where you come upon a roadblock and have to ram through it in order to save your life. Hopefully, you'll never have to do this. A few things to know about ramming cars. Hollywood gets this totally wrong. You cannot ram a car as you're traveling down the highway at 60 miles per hour. Going this fast can disable the car you're in, and you'll never be able to speed away once you get through the roadblock. In fact, you want to be going 20 to 25 miles per hour—tops. Not only is this the right speed for moving the other car but it ensures that the car you are driving will keep running. You also want to aim to hit the other car just to the right of the gas tank—toward the back. You don't want to hit the car up front where the engine is—it's too heavy.

1. Approach the vehicle going at least (but not much more than) 20 miles per hour. If for someone reason you hit your brakes and you're trying to ram a car at 5 miles per hour, you won't move the car, but will basically just have had a minor car accident.
2. Hit the car at the back of the vehicle near the gas tank. Don't forget to keep your foot on the gas and acceler-

ate through the vehicle. In other words, keep your foot on the gas pedal the entire time as you're ramming the vehicle and don't lift it off as you drive through the vehicle.

3. Once the car has moved out of your way, continue driving, speeding up as necessary to escape.

The Down Driver

Have you ever thought about what you would do if the person who was driving you in a car was shot in an ambush—or perhaps more likely, has a heart attack? There is a simple way to handle this situation should it ever happen to you.

1. Your driver is down. Grab onto either the back of the seat, or the handle above the driver's-side window so that you have some leverage.
2. Bring your right leg or left leg (whichever works better for you) over to the driver's side and use it to operate the gas pedal. If you need to, push the driver's leg to the side.
3. Drive to safety.

Again, I hope you never need to use any of these evasive driving maneuvers in real life, but since this world is so unpredictable you just never know.

12

DEFENDING YOURSELF

Weapons and Important Self-Defense Tactics

Bruce Lee, one of the most famous martial artists of all time, said, "I fear not the man who has practiced 10,000 kicks one time, but I fear the man who has practiced one kick 10,000 times." Mastering self-defense tactics isn't about knowing everything—it's about being good at a few simple techniques, so that in the event you use them, you can execute them flawlessly. Many of the situations I'm going to describe in this chapter can be handled using very similar techniques. I highly recommend that you practice these techniques for two minutes each day. If you commit to practicing just two minutes a day, you'll eventually find that you can execute these maneuvers without even thinking about it. Just pick one to start with and move onto a new one once you feel comfortable with it. While I hope you never encounter a dangerous situation, the skills you learn in this chapter could save your life or the life of a loved one.

Escape to Gain Safety

Even though I'm a very capable guy—I train six days a week—I'm never going to put myself in a situation where I have to fight. I would always make a point to deescalate and would use these tactics only if I really had to. Also know that the goal is for you to create a situation in which you can escape and get help. While it could be necessary to keep throwing punches or stab someone, if the situation allows, it's always better to escape and get help.

 It's always better to escape and get help.

The acronym ETGS (escape to gain safety) will help you remember what to do if you are being attacked. These principles can be used in most of the scenarios I talk about in this chapter:

E   *escape = eyes: You can gouge or poke the attacker's eyes.*
T   *to = throat: You can strike the attacker in the throat, larynx, or voice box. A hit here will cause the person to stumble backward.*
G   *gain = groin: If the attacker is in front of you, kick the person in the groin.*
S   *safety = shin: You can kick the attacker repeatedly in the shin. If the person is wearing shorts, you can rub your foot hard against the skin.*

I'm going to go over how to deal with some serious situations, should they ever come up. However, the most important things to remember are to *get off the X, do not freeze,* and as you'll see, *control*

the threat. Once you've accomplished this, your number one priority in any emergency situation is to get away and get help.

The Situation: Someone Grabs Your Arm and Is Going to Drag You

It is essential that you teach this tactic to your kids—everyone in
your family should know what to do if someone grabs your arm
and tries to drag you off somewhere. The first thing you need to
do is fight. Although the natural reaction is to step back, stepping
back is just going to put you in a tug of war with the attacker. Instead, you want to step in, abruptly bringing your elbow up and in
toward the attacker's face. Thrusting your elbow up will break the
lock he's got on your arm, and you can escape to safety. You can
see a video of me demonstrating this at SpySecretsBook.com.

For Small Children
If we're dealing with small children, or just a very strong attacker,
there's one added element that will break the hold. If you cannot
bring your arm up to break the attacker's hold, bring your opposite
hand over to grab onto the arm the attacker is holding. The additional leverage from your opposite arm will help break the hold.

The Situation: You're Grabbed from Behind in a Bear Hug

You're jogging along your favorite path when someone jumps out
of the bushes and grabs you in a bear hug. In this instance, instead
of trying to run forward, take a large step backward to throw the

attacker off balance. At the same time, you're going to start peeling away fingers, potentially breaking them. Little ones are especially easy to damage. Eventually, after you've done enough damage to the hands, the attacker will let go. At this point, you can do an elbow to the neck, or reach back and hit the groin and then run to safety.

If the Attacker Tries to Elevate You

If your attacker tries to elevate you by leaning back and lifting you up, hook your leg behind his, which will keep him from getting a good grip on you. Then the technique is the same as if you get grabbed in a bear hug. Start breaking away at the fingers until the attacker lets go and you can escape.

The Situation: An Attacker Grabs Your Hair

While this is something women need to worry about more than men, just know that it's still possible to grab someone by the hair even if it's very short. If someone approaches you from the front and grabs your hair, know that he is actually placing himself in a good position for you to attack back. And because he's in front of you, you know exactly what the attacker is doing. You also know that he can't attack you with the hand that's holding your hair. In this situation, you're going to remember what we talked about in the beginning of the chapter: escape to gain safety. In this instance, the letters in the acronym give you the clues about what to do. Because the attacker is in front of you, you can attack back with a barrage of hits. Remember ETGS: eyes, throat, groin, and shins.

Once you've thrown a barrage of strikes at the attacker and

have broken free, run to a populated area, making as much noise as you possibly can.

Your Hair Is Grabbed from Behind

While you can't see your attacker in this situation, you still know exactly where he is. It's important not to pull away from your attacker. Instead, reach up and grab his hands, holding him as tightly to you as possible. Begin to rotate, still holding him tightly, until you see that his arm is bent backward. At this point you can peel his hands off, strike using ETGS, and run away.

The Situation: Someone Has You in a Choke Hold

While someone trying to choke you is obviously a serious situation you'd need to get out of immediately, this technique will also work if someone is just grabbing onto your shirt in a threatening way. This technique is incredibly simple, but effective. To make sure you know how to execute this if you ever need it, note the space on your neck where there is an indentation. It's very sensitive, and that's where you're going to hit your attacker. When the person's hands hit your neck, simply jab two fingers quickly and firmly into the indentation in her neck. I guarantee you, the person is going to gag, her chin will go down, and she'll step backward, giving you an opportunity to escape.

The Situation: Someone Is Going to Punch You

So what do you do if you encounter someone who looks like he's going to hit you? I personally always keep my hands up whenever someone enters my personal space, just to stay aware and be ready. I'm not going to do this in a threatening way—I don't want to escalate a situation by acting threatening. You're basically putting up a barrier so you can react quickly if you need to. Let's say some guy throws one of those big, roundhouse punches your way—like he's trying to knock your head off. What you're going to do is keep your arms bent upward, so that you can crash into his upper arm when he throws the punch. Now you're in a good position to turn toward the attacker and hack him in the neck. At this point you can engage or run to safety. This technique puts you in a good position to hit your attacker at the occipital notch, or the spot at the back of the head where the spine meets the skull. It should be noted that a slap at the occipital notch is extremely disorienting.

If the Punch Is Straight On

The technique you'll use if a punch comes straight at you is slightly different. If you feel threatened, you'll want your arms up (again, don't aggravate the situation by putting your arms up in a threatening way), elevated to about shoulder height. When the punch comes straight at you, you'll bend your forearms up so that the punch lands right on the tip of your elbow.

Hitting your elbow hard is really going to hurt your attacker— this maneuver can easily end up breaking fingers. If you wanted to imagine what this feels like, think about how it would feel if you were to make a fist and punch the corner of your dining room table as hard as you could. Once the attacker has hit your elbow, or possibly broken fingers, you can use some of the moves from the ETGS principles or simply run to safety.

What You Need to Know About Choosing and Using Weapons

The Tactical Pen

As I mentioned in Chapter 3, the tactical pen is one of my favorite things to carry. You can take it absolutely everywhere (including airplanes), and it's a good option for those of you who don't feel ready to carry a knife or a gun or who live somewhere where you are prohibited from doing so. The tactical pen I use looks harmless enough, but if you examine it more closely you'll notice it has some features that your average pen doesn't have. It's much thicker and heavier than a regular pen (it's made of aircraft-grade aluminum), but most important, the bottom end of the pen has a sharp point. Don't worry, it's not so sharp that you'll be cut if you reach into your purse or laptop bag to get it—but you can do serious damage with that end of the pen. In the class I teach about defending yourself with a tactical pen, I always demonstrate how tough these pens are by hammering one into a block of ice. A regular pen just gets crushed—but with just a couple of hits with the hammer, the tactical pen I use actually splits a block of ice right in half. These pens are strong. Not only can you hurt an attacker by stabbing or jabbing at him with a pen, but you could also use it to break glass in an emergency.

The Right Tactical Pen

I've tested out every tactical pen that's out there, and my favorite costs $35.00 (they range from $10.00 to as much as $300). You can see the tactical pen I use at TacticalSpyPen.com. Whatever pen you decide to buy, make sure you consider the following:

- Buy quality (this is a rule of thumb for all weapons).
- It should have a solid metal point for striking.
- It should have a clip on it to clip to your pants pocket or inside your pants. (It won't do you any good if it's laying on the bottom of your purse or briefcase.)
- It should have a flat cap end to allow for a solid grip and so you can place your thumb on the cap for extra striking power.
- It must write well and have refillable ink so you can use it for a very long time.

The Grip

The first thing you need to know about defending yourself with a tactical pen is how to grip the pen properly. It's possible to use the underhand grip. Think of the underhand grip as if you were holding a sword and you were jabbing it at someone. However, you'll see that with this grip, you don't actually have a great deal of leverage. It's going to be harder to do serious damage this way. Or you can use the icepick grip (also known as the reverse grip). The ice pick grip gives you more control over the pen and more power when striking. As I just mentioned, you want to have your thumb on top of the pen so that you have more support.

Where to Carry Your Tactical Pen

This is very important. Your tactical pen must be accessible if it's going to be useful. You don't want to be digging around for it if you find yourself in a dangerous situation. I like to carry my tactical pen clipped to the inside of my right front pants pocket. It works for me, and I always know where to reach for it should I need to use it. Wherever you decide to carry it, keep it consistent. You need to develop muscle memory so that you automatically know where to reach for it. Some places you can clip your pen and still have it be accessible are a pants pocket, a T-shirt collar, a purse strap, or the inside of your pants.

Deploying the Pen

This is a simple three-step process:

1. Get a grip on the pen.
2. Draw the pen straight up.
3. Drive the pen straight out (almost like you were drawing a gun).

It's good to practice deploying your tactical pen as if you were in a variety of threatening situations. Practice drawing your pen quickly in a variety of simulated situations—standing, on your back, while walking, while stepping off line (or off the X), if someone has you in a bear hug, or if there's a person walking up to you. If you can't get your pen up and out from any of these positions, you need to find a different place to carry your pen. A great way to practice is by having a friend or family member hold up a used pizza box. Practice drawing your pen up and out, and striking the box.

Using Your Tactical Pen to Deflect a Punch

We've already gone over how to defend yourself if someone throws a punch at you, but the tactical pen adds an additional element. Should you be in a place where you feel uncomfortable— you're walking through a rough neighborhood or you're in a bar or restaurant and someone's looking at you funny—get out your tactical pen. Since you always want to deescalate a situation, you don't want to be holding it in a threatening manner. You should hold it discreetly in your hand, letting it rest on your forearm so the potential attacker can't see it. If the attacker throws a big roundhouse punch at you, use the technique I described earlier, raising your arm up to block the punch. However, use your other hand—the one holding the tactical pen—to reach out and firmly jab your attacker in the armpit or pectoral muscles. This is going to hurt.

If the Punch Comes Straight at You

Again, you'll use the same technique as you would if someone were throwing a punch straight at you. In this case, however, you'll rotate the hand with the tactical pen upward, so that the attacker's punch lands right on the tip of your pen. As you might imagine, this is not going to feel good.

Carrying a Knife: What You Need to Know

As always, you need to be familiar with what's legal to carry in your state. Make sure you investigate the legality of carrying a knife where you live *before* you start carrying one. As with most things, you need to find out what works for you. There are a few things you'll want to consider before you buy a knife:

- Where are you going to carry it? On your belt? In your pocket?
- What kind of clothes do you wear? If you wear jeans most days, you can manage a knife with a rougher edge. If you

Don't Forget About Deployment

Most people don't practice this, but it's crucial to know how to properly get your knife out and into action. Make sure you learn the proper technique for deploying your knife from a trained professional. Deploying your knife should feel like second nature and should be something you don't have to think twice about should you be involved in an attack.

wear suits, you're going to rip the fabric and you'll need a knife with a smoother handle.

- How will you deploy the knife? Manually, or do you want an automatic opener?
- How heavy can it be?
- How big can it be?

It's important that you select a knife that you are comfortable carrying with you *every* day. Be consistent. In an emergency situation, you don't want to have to pause and think, "What knife am I carrying today?" You want to know what you have on you at all times and how to deploy it.

Step Off the *X* in a Knife Attack

We're going to look at some basic footwork that moves you off the *X* should you be attacked by someone with a knife. Good knife defense training is based on triangles; it's all angular movements. The only time you would ever move straight forward in an engagement is if you are pushing someone back very hard in a knife attack.

The Footwork Matrix

If you want to practice this move, you can place electrical tape on your floor. You'll want to make a big letter *X*, with a horizontal line through the middle. It's like you're taping a huge asterisk onto the ground. This provides some guidance for when you're practicing stepping off the *X* for all of the following movements, whether you are advancing, retreating, or sidestepping.

The Forward Triangle

The forward triangle opens you up because you are stepping off the line to one side while you're advancing forward. You're taking a forty-five-degree step in relation to the oncoming threat. This move is very simple. If you want to move left, your left leg is going to step off the line first. If moving to the right, your right leg moves first. You would step to the side that is *zoning you away from the threat*. This move is putting you in a position to avoid incoming damage from the attacker. Your footwork brings you in, to where you can do damage, and then back out, to avoid damage. An added benefit to this movement is that it puts you in a position to use your hips for more power if you need to hit your attacker hard. Just keep in mind that you want to remain in balance as you move back and forth in this fashion.

Backward Movement

You can also move backward from the center in the same forty-five-degree angle to keep yourself away from the threat. You just need to practice moving your body comfortably forward and backward, getting used to the way the movements feel. Should you encounter a threat, you won't have time to think about which way to go.

Sideways Move and Pivot

You can also move from side to side if the threat is coming at you directly from the front. Step to the side and pivot, rotating your body quickly to the back.

Learn More About Knife Defense

Learning to defend yourself with a knife is serious business that requires skill and practice. I highly recommend that if you'd like to learn more about knife skills, that you check out my training at TwoSecondSurvival.com and find a reputable training center in your area. This training can provide serious peace of mind—as you'll know exactly what to do in the event that you find a knife at your back while at the ATM or a knife at your throat while someone is trying to steal your car. Proper knife training will also teach you how to do the following:

- Disarm an attacker with a knife whether the knife is at your throat, chest, or back.

What Does a Former CIA Officer Do to Stay in Shape?

People expect that a former CIA officer has a workout routine worthy of Rambo.

The truth is my workout is much simpler than that—but very effective. Anyone can do it. I wish I were the kind of person who loved running or working out, but I'm not. I do it out of necessity, for several reasons. I'll start with the extreme scenarios of why I believe you need to be in shape. If there's an end of the world situation or a natural disaster I want to be able to flee on foot without getting tired after ten steps. If I have to walk several miles with my seventy-two-hour kit on my back, I don't want to have any problem with the extra twenty-two pounds I'm carrying.

I also want to be able to flee in a short-term crisis situation. If I'm ever in a parking lot and someone pulls a knife on me or points a gun at me, I want to be able to quickly move out of the line of fire and defend myself. Or what if you're at the mall and you hear gunshots from the other end of the mall where your spouse or kids happen to be shopping? You obviously want to be able to make it to the other end of the mall as fast as possible without giving yourself a heart attack.

This simple workout routine will give you the explosive power to move fast in an emergency situation.

Monday: I do a high intensity workout. I sprint hard for fifteen to thirty seconds and then take a sixty-second break. And when I say sprint hard, I mean it. You're giving it everything you've got for those fifteen to thirty seconds and if you're not huffing and puffing and feeling like you want to die then you're not pushing yourself hard enough. I do this five times and then take a half-mile walk to cool down.

Tuesday: I go for an easy two-and-a-half-mile run. I'm jogging during this run and not killing myself, but I'm breaking a good sweat.

Wednesday: Another high-intensity training day. Five fifteen-to thirty-second sprints with a sixty-second resting period after each one. Cool down with a half-mile walk.

Thursday: Another long run, jogging for two and a half miles.

Friday: Another high-intensity day, the same routine I do on Monday and Wednesday.

Obviously, you can modify it however you wish. But if you haven't done any type of exercising in a long time, I would consider changing that tomorrow. If you're like me, it won't be the most fun thing in the world, but your body will thank you for it. And you'll have peace of mind, knowing that if a crisis should arise, you'll be better physically prepared to flee to safety.

- Disarm an attacker who is carjacking you using the leverage from your steering wheel.
- Disarm an attacker who may have been hiding in the backseat of your car—this is possible to do even if your car is moving.

- Disarm an attacker who has invaded your home while you were sleeping and has a knife to your throat.
- How to attack someone in lethal force situations using vital targets, such as the brachial artery, the internal jugular, and the heart, and disembowelment.

Acknowledgments

I'm extremely grateful to so many people who made this book possible. I'd like to thank ████████████████████████ for the fun times we had. Don't get yourself killed wherever you are these days. And I can't forget ███████████████████ who ██████████ ██. There's also ██████████ and ███████████ whose crazy ██████████████████████ made all of this possible. And last, but certainly not least, I'd like to thank ████████████. Remember the time we ███████████████████. What a fun ride we had doing ██████████████████████. And to everyone else reading this, thank you and keep yourselves safe.

References

Aldax, Mike. "Texting While Walking around San Francisco? Watch for Muggers." *San Francisco Examiner*, February 3, 2011.

"American Serial Killer and Rapist Ted Bundy Was One of the Most Notorious Criminals of the Late 20th Century." *Bio*, A&E Networks Television, 2015.

"Armed Man Robs Senior Couple at Knifepoint in Hyannis Hotel Room." CBS Boston, September 1, 2014.

"Attempted Kidnapping Thwarted in Downtown Redding, Police Say." *Record Searchlight*, May 8, 2014.

Balkenbush, Molly. "Woman Claims Cab Driver Robbed, Raped Her." Fox 4 Kansas City, October 1, 2014.

Barnes, Iris. "Bank Robbery and Fake Bomb Threats Are Connected, According to Grenada Police." NewsMs., September 8, 2014.

Bauer, Jennifer. "Officials: Woman Carjacked at Stoplight." Click2Houston, October 22, 2012.

Bearman, Joshuah. "How the CIA Used a Fake Sci-Fi Flick to Rescue Americans from Tehran." *Wired*, April 24, 2007.

Bellware, Kim. "Bogus Chicago Taxi Driver Scams Chinese Student Out of $4,240 in Cab Ride Ruse." *Huffington Post*, September 3, 2013.

Benjamin, Kathy. "60% of People Can't Go 10 Minutes Without Lying." Mental Floss, May 7, 2012.

Bennett, Erica. "Neighbor Spots Potential Burglar Parked Outside Orange Park Home." CBS 47 Jacksonville, July 7, 2014.

Bennhold, Katrin. "Years of Rape and 'Utter Contempt' in Britain." *New York Times*, September 1, 2014.

Bentz, Leslie. "Report: Naked Woman Distracts Man as Her Accomplice Robs His House." CNN, July 10, 2013.

Bloxham, Andy. "British Students Gang Raped on Caribbean Island." *Telegraph (UK)*, May 18, 2011.

"Bronx Woman Followed Home, Sexually Assaulted, Police Search for Suspect." ABC 7 Los Angeles, October 3, 2013.

Boyle, Louise. "Girl, 15, Crushed to Death by Truck After She Stumbled Off Curb While Distracted by Her Phone." *Daily Mail (UK)*. January 31, 2014.

Brumfield, Ben, and Steve Almasy. "Passengers Cry and Pray as Smoke-Filled Plane Rattles to Emergency Landing." CNN, September 19, 2014.

Bucktin, Christopher. "Terrifying Photo Shows Woman Hiding on Roof from Intruder—Then He Appears Behind Her." *Daily Mirror (UK)*, September 25, 2014.

"Capturing Whitey Bulger: How the FBI Finally Caught Up with the Country's No.1 Most Wanted . . . and It Was All Thanks to a Boob Job and a Stray Cat." *Daily Mail (UK)*, November 25, 2013.

"Car Found After Woman Beaten, Carjacked at Phipps Plaza." WSB-TV 2 Atlanta, August 5, 2014.

Carrascco, Tracee. "Mysterious Tape or Delivery Slip on Your Home? It Could Be Burglars Doing Recon." CBS New York, July 24, 2014.

"Cary Police Seek Sexual Assault Suspect." *Raleigh (NC) News & Observer*, April 14, 2014.

Chin, Alyssa. "Car Stolen While Left Warming Up." KKTV 11, Colorado Springs/Pueblo, January 5, 2014.

Christian, Susan. "Burning Memories: Ten Years Later, Survivors Continue to Relive the MGM Grand Fire. 'Once You've Been Through an Experience Like That, It Stays with You Forever.'" *Los Angeles Times*, November 18, 1990.

"Cops: Fake Cabbie Tries to Rape Woman in Front of Kids in New York City." *Crimesider*, CBS News, August 28, 2014.

Counts, John. "Police Arrest Ann Arbor Man They Believe Attempted to Sexually Assault U-M Student." MLive Michigan, May 8, 2014.

"Couple Robbed by 3 Men in Md. Hotel Room." WUSA 9 Washington, DC, October 1, 2012.

Courtenay-Smith, Natasha. "I Lost Three Best Friends and Almost Died in the Tsunami . . . How Could My Husband Then Walk Out on Me?" *Daily Mail (UK)*, December 24, 2009.

"Crimetracker: Wanted Suspects Faked Car Trouble, Robbed Victims." WVLT Knoxville, May 13, 2013.

"Crying Woman Tricks Tourists into Opening Motel Door." WFTV 9 Orlando, May 19, 2009.

Dewan, Shaila, and Janet Roberts. "Louisiana's Deadly Storm Took Strong as Well as Helpless." *New York Times*, December 18, 2005.

Diaz, Mario. "Man Charged in SI Home Invasion That Left Elderly Man Dead, Wife Injured." WPIX TV New York, September 1, 2014.

Dowling, Courtney. "We Survived Two Home Invasions in Three Years." Insight Orlando, May 6, 2014.

Ellison, Annie. "Woman Recalls Being Kidnapped by Kelly Swoboda." KOIN Portland, April 30, 2014.

Fasick, Kevin, and Kevin Sheehan. "Busted NJ Carjack Suspects Have Long Rap Sheets." *New York Post*, December 21, 2013.

Fernandez, Manny, and Alison Leigh Cowan. "When Horror Came to a Connecticut Family." *New York Times*, August 6, 2007.

"The Fire This Time." *People*, February 25, 1991.

Fleece, Larry, and Chip Yost. "San Clemente 'Distraction' Robbery Nets $200,000." KTLA Los Angeles, January 10, 2013.

Freund, Helen. "Reserve Couple's Bodies Were Bound by Rope, One to Kettlebell, Police Say." *New Orleans Times-Picayune*, April 2, 2014.

Frick Carlman, Susan. "Erin Sarris: 'I Knew Something Was Wrong.'" *Naperville Sun*, April 19, 2014.

"Fugitive Doctor Gets Prison for Massive Patient Fraud." *New York Daily News*, October 13, 2012.

"Fugitives from Colorado Springs Arrested in Walsenburg After Crash." KKTV Colorado Springs/Pueblo, January 9, 2014.

George, Justin. "Many Vehicles Stolen in Baltimore Are Left Running, Police Say." *Baltimore Sun*, July 19, 2014.

Goldstein, Joseph. "At Manhattan Restaurant, a Robbery and an Oblivious Customer." *New York Times*, September 15, 2014.

Goldstein, Sasha. "Ala. Man Runs over, Kills Grandmother as Horrified Daughter, Grandson Watch: Police." *New York Daily News*, June 27, 2014.

Goodnough, Abby. "Crime Boss in Hiding Found Time for Travels." *New York Times*, June 27, 2011.

Grimm, Andy. "Nearly 7 Years for Sinus Doctor in Medical Fraud." *Chicago Tribune*, October 12, 2012.

Harshbarger, Rebecca, and Bob Fredericks. "Texting Comic Run Over by Train Finds the Funny Side." *New York Post*, February 14, 2014.

Hasnie, Aishah. "Don't Ignore Door Knock, Says Sheriff after Attempted Break-in." Fox 59 Indianapolis, August 28, 2014.

Heath, Brad. "The Ones That Get Away." *USA Today*, October 21, 2014.

Hobson, Alex. "Two Tampa Teens Found Dead, Tied Together, on Road in Jacksonville." WFTS Tampa Bay, September 18, 2014.

Holliday, Ian. "'I Was Furious': Good Samaritan Duped by Scam Artists." CTV News Vancouver, July 8, 2014.

Hopper, Brandi. "Police: 'Polite' Home Invasion Suspects Entered through Open Garage Door." Fox 59 Indianapolis, December 18, 2013.

Hruby, Patrick. "Ex-CIA Disguise Experts Putting a Human Face on Oft-maligned U.S. Spies." *Washington Times*, September 27, 2011.

Huber, Mark. "How Things Work: Evacuation Slides." *Air & Space*, November 2007.

"'I Knew Something Was Terribly Wrong.'" NPR, September 29 2013.

Irby, Kate. "Suspect Impersonating Police Officer Tells Bradenton Woman to Get in His Car." *Bradenton (FL) Herald*, September 15, 2014.

Jefferson, Steve. "Cars Stolen, Woman Shot during Indianapolis Home Invasion." WTHR 13 Indianapolis, October 29, 2013.

"Judge Rules Scott Peterson to Stand Trial." CNN, January 7, 2004.

Kamm, Grayson. "Nurse Carjacked While Reading Bible." 11 Alive Atlanta, June 3, 2014.

Klimas, Liz. "Good Samaritan's Selfless Act Ends with a Gun to His Family's Head." *Blaze*, November 6, 2013.

Lawrence, Tom. "Rescued . . . Family Trapped in Snow Tomb for 2 Days." *Daily Express (UK)*, December 24, 2011.

Lehman, Pamela. "Springfield Township Police Said Woman Robbed of Jewelry and Rifle in Distraction Burglary." *Allentown (PA) Morning Call*, July 17, 2014.

Lohr, David. "Carlesha Freeland-Gaither Missing: Shocking Video of Woman's Abduction." *Huffington Post*, November 4, 2014.

Lohr, David. "Christopher Newsom, Channon Christian Remembered, 6 Years after Horrific Torture Slaying." *Huffington Post*, January 7, 2013.

"Man Impersonating Officer in Manatee." WTSP 10 News Tampa Bay, September 15, 2014.

Mann, Zarni. "Passengers Had 90 Seconds to Escape Crashed Plane." *Irrawaddy*, December 27, 2012.

Matas, Kimberly. "3 Men Arrested in Deadly Tucson Home Invasion." *Arizona Daily Star*, October 7, 2014.

Mazzetti, Mark, Helene Cooper, and Peter Baker. "Behind the Hunt for Bin Laden." *New York Times*, May 2, 2011.

Medina, Jennifer, and Ian Lovett. "Bulger's Neighbors Knew a 'Nice' Couple Who Took Walks." *New York Times*, June 23, 2011.

Milligan, Susan. "The Trouble with Uber." *U.S. News & World Report*, July 15, 2014.

Moffet, Penelope. "Jet Crash Lingers in Memory: Survivor Recalls Horror of Disaster That Killed 582." *Los Angeles Times*, March 27, 1987.

Moore, Tina, Ryan Sit, and Corky Siemaszko. "Short Hills Carjacking Victim Died Defending Wife." *New York Daily News*, December 16, 2013.

Moran, Lee. "Teen Rams Vehicle into Police Car during Kidnap Attempt." *New York Daily News*, March 27, 2013.

Moskowitz, Eric. "Carjack Victim Recounts His Harrowing Night." *Boston Globe*, April 25, 2013.

Nagourney, Adam, and Ian Lovett. "Whitey Bulger Is Arrested in California." *New York Times*, June 22, 2011.

Neuhauser, Alan. "Scam Artists Targeting Asian Tourists in Wine-Bottle Ruse, Police Warn." DNAinfo: New York, March 26, 2013.

Nuzzi, Olivia. "Uber's Biggest Problem Isn't Surge Pricing. What If It's Sexual Harassment by Drivers?" *Daily Beast*, March 28, 2014.

"NYC: Taxi Drivers' Meter Scam Bilked Riders Out of $8.3M-Plus." *USA Today*, March 13, 2010.

Nye, James. "Almost Famous! Student Hired Own Bodyguards, Paparazzi and Entourage and Pranked New York into Believing He Was a World-Famous Celebrity." *Daily Mail (UK)*, August 24, 2012.

O'Riordan, Sean. "'Reconnaissance Units' Stake Out Houses for Burglar Gangs." *Irish Examiner*, April 10, 2013.

"Oregon Sicko Who Stalked Women from 'Moveable Dungeon' Died in Shootout." *New York Daily News*, April 22, 2014.

Ortega, Ralph R., and Rick Hepp. "Trucker Tells How He Killed Woman in Bloomsbury." *Newark Star-Ledger*, October 4, 2008.

Padilla, Cecilio. "Physician Assistant Allegedly Rigs Car for Kidnappings and Rapes." FOX 40 Sacramento, October 9, 2013.

Pangyanszki, Jennifer. "3 Days of Death, Despair and Survival." CNN, September 9, 2005.

Papenfuss, Mary. "Laci Hubby in Wacky Makeover: New Hair & Beard—Plus Eye for Border?" *New York Daily News*, April 20, 2003.

Parascandola, Rocco, and Kerry Willis. "Hunt 3 in Savage Bx. Slaying." *New York Daily News*, December 21, 2011.

Patel, Tina. "Driver: Brazen Thief Reached in, Stole iPad While I Was Meditating in Car." Fox News, September 9, 2014.

Pawula, Larissa. "The Smart Murder." *Portsmouth Herald*, March 27, 1991.

Perleberg, Mike. "Stranded Motorist Twice Scams Good Samaritan." *Eagle Country Online*, March 21, 2014.

Persley, Mike. "Fake Taxi Driver Pleads Guilty to Scam, Stealing More Than $200,000." *DC Inno*, August 4, 2014.

Pesta, Abigail. "The Day My Husband Disappeared." *Marie Claire*, March 15, 2011.

Pierson Curtis, Henry. "Four Teen Girls Rob and Ram Victim to Party." *Orlando Sentinel*, March 5, 2012.

Pierson Curtis, Henry. "Tourist Shot in Hotel Robbery." *Orlando Sentinel*, October 6, 1992.

"Police Find Stolen Car with 2-Year-Old Boy Inside." CBS Minnesota, September 25, 2014.

"Police ID Suspect Who Posed as UPS Driver, Tied Up and Robbed Elderly Woman." KMOV 4 St. Louis, May 28, 2013.

Rennell, Tony. "'I Breathed Water and, Oh God, the Panic . . . Then the Tsunami Tore My Daughter from My Arms.'" *Daily Mail (UK)*, December 19, 2009.

Rowson, Kevin. "Georgia Good Samaritan Scammed by Couple She Helped." *USA Today*, May 13, 2014.

Ruiz, Travis. "WANTED: Armed and Dangerous Home Burglars in Colorado Springs." Fox 21 Colorado Springs, January 3, 2014.

Sacks, Ethan. "Intruder Breaks into Mike Tyson's Hotel Room." *New York Daily News*, January 5, 2012.

Santora, Marc, and Annie Correal. "Man Dies in Carjacking at Short Hills Mall; 2 Suspects Are Sought." *New York Times*, December 16, 2013.

Santora, Marc. "A Knock on the Door, a Stranger, Then a Killing at a Rural Summer Home." *New York Times*, August 25, 2014.

Santora, Marc. "Man, 20, Is Charged With Fatal Stabbing in S. I. Home Invasion." *New York Times*, September 1, 2014.

Satterfield, Jamie, and Don Jacobs. "Details of Double Slaying Emerge." *Knoxville News Sentinel*, January 13, 2007.

Scott, Luci. "Gilbert School's Tiger Mascot Ignites Roar of Crowd." *Arizona Republic*, February 18, 2013.

Seltzer, Alexandra. "Police Say 'Bump and Rob' Crime Is Back, Ask Public to Be Aware of Surroundings." *Palm Beach Post*, March 6, 2014.

Sharot, Tali. "The Optimism Bias." *Time*, May 28, 2011.

"Southwest Flight Makes Emergency Landing at LAX." *USA Today*, September 21, 2014.

Sullivan, Randall. "The World's Best Bounty Hunter Is 4-Foot-11. Here's How She Hunts." *Wired*, December 17, 2013.

Swalec, Andrew. "Armed Robber in FedEx Jacket Hits Thompson Street Apartment." DNAinfo: New York, January 6, 2012.

Terruso, Julia. "Man Charged in Millburn Video Attack Committed Similar Offense 20 Years Ago." *Newark Star-Ledger,* July 2, 2013.

"Toledo, Ohio, Officials Warn against Drinking Toxic Tap Water." CBS News, August 2, 2014.

Tuttle, Brad. "There's Just No Stopping Las Vegas Taxi Drivers from Overcharging Tourists." *Time,* February 26, 2014.

U.S. Department of Justice. "Carjacking, 1993–2002." Crime Data Brief, July 2004.

Vedantam, Shankar. "The Decoy Effect, or How to Win an Election." *Washington Post,* April 2, 2007.

Villalon, Debora. "Target Employee Pivotal in Finding Abducted Child: 'I Knew Something Was Wrong,'" Fox News Latino, January 8, 2014.

Werbach, Adam, and Saba Hamedy. "The American Commuter Spends 38 Hours a Year Stuck in Traffic." *Atlantic,* February 6, 2013.

Whitlock, Craig, and Barton Gellman. "To Hunt Osama Bin Laden, Satellites Watched over Abbottabad, Pakistan, and Navy SEALs." *Washington Post,* August 29, 2013.

"Why We Think Ignorance Is Bliss, Even When It Hurts Our Health." NPR, July 23, 2014.

Williams, David. "Drivers Urged to Be Aware of Potential Car-Theft Scam." *Telegraph (UK),* November 11 2009.

"Woman Carjacked at Red Light in Flint." MLive Michigan, August 11, 2011.

Yaniv, Oren. "Taxi Driver Gets 20 Years for Raping Passenger." *New York Daily News,* May 12, 2014.

Zucchino, David, and Lisa Mascaro. "Snowed-In Atlanta: Drivers Trapped Overnight; Kids Sleep at School." *Los Angeles Times,* January 29, 2014.

Index

About the Author

Jason R. Hanson is a former CIA officer, security specialist, and winner on ABC's hit reality series *Shark Tank*. Jason has appeared on the *Today Show* and *Dateline* and is a frequent guest on the *Rachael Ray Show*. Jason has been interviewed by major media outlets for his security expertise, including the *Wall Street Journal*, Fox News, *Forbes*, NPR, and the *Huffington Post*. He advises Fortune 500 companies on their security protocols and runs an executive protection and investigations firm. He currently lives in Cedar City, Utah, with his family.